# 海关卫生检疫

## 常用英语场景会话手册

本书编委会 编著

中国海关出版社有限公司

中国·北京

**图书在版编目（CIP）数据**

海关卫生检疫常用英语场景会话手册 / 本书编委会编著 . -- 北京 : 中国海关出版社有限公司 , 2024. 11.
ISBN 978-7-5175-0848-9

Ⅰ . R185.3-62

中国国家版本馆 CIP 数据核字第 202462X0B5 号

## 海关卫生检疫常用英语场景会话手册

HAIGUAN WEISHENG JIANYI CHANGYONG YINGYU CHANGJING HUIHUA SHOUCE

作　　者：本书编委会
责任编辑：夏淑婷
责任印制：孙　倩
出版发行：中国海关出版社有限公司
社　　址：北京市朝阳区东四环南路甲 1 号　　邮政编码：100023
编 辑 部：01065194242-7539（电话）
发 行 部：01065194221/4238/4246/5127（电话）
社办书店：01065195616（电话）
https: //weidian.com/? userid=319526934（网址）
印　　刷：北京金康利印刷有限公司　　经　　销：新华书店
开　　本：710mm × 1000mm　1/16
印　　张：14　　字　　数：262 千字
版　　次：2024 年 11 月第 1 版
印　　次：2024 年 11 月第 1 次印刷
书　　号：ISBN 978-7-5175-0848-9
定　　价：88.00 元

# 本书编委会

# 前言

为了提高卫生检疫人员的英语水平，加强卫生检疫工作，本书编委会组织厦门海关卫生检疫相关领域专家编写了《海关卫生检疫常用英语场景会话手册》，供卫生检疫人员在工作中参考。

本书按照入境人员卫生检疫、入境交通工具卫生检疫、突发公共卫生事件应急处置、国际旅行健康服务四个方面，设计了多个会话场景，力求专业知识准确、语言描述精练。希望本书的出版对提高卫生检疫人员工作技能水平，筑牢国门生物安全屏障，保障人民群众身体健康有所裨益。

由于编者水平有限，书中难免有疏漏之处，敬请专家和广大读者批评指正！

本书编委会

2024 年 9 月

# 目录

CONTENTS

## 第一章　入境人员卫生检疫

CHAPTER I　HEALTH QUARANTINE OF ENTRY PERSONNEL

## 第二章　入境交通工具卫生检疫
## CHAPTER II　HEALTH QUARANTINE OF INBOUND VEHICLES

### 第一部分　航空器登临检疫
### PART I　BOARDING AND QUARANTINE OF AIRCRAFT

# 第三章 突发公共卫生事件应急处置
# CHAPTER III RESPONDING TO A PUBLIC HEALTH EMERGENCY

## 第一部分 船舶（货轮）
## PART I SHIPS (CARGO SHIPS)

# 第二部分 邮轮消化道疾病聚集性暴发事件应急处置

PART II RESPONDING TO THE OUTBREAK OF A CLUSTER OF GASTROINTESTINAL INFECTIONS ON A CRUISE SHIP

## 第四章 国际旅行健康服务
CHAPTER IV HEALTH SERVICES FOR INTERNATIONAL TRAVELERS

## 附 录 APPENDIX

# 第一章

CHAPTER I

# 入境人员卫生检疫

HEALTH QUARANTINE OF ENTRY PERSONNEL

## 第一节 健康申报
## SECTION I HEALTH DECLARATION

**检疫关员：**您好，请问有什么能帮您的？

Officer: Hello, can I help you?

**旅客：**我有一点头晕和咳嗽。

Passenger: I had a little bit dizziness and coughing.

**检疫关员：**请出示您的护照和健康申明卡。

Officer:Please show me your passport and Health Declaration Form.

**旅客：**好的，这是护照，但是我还没有填写健康申明卡。

Passenger: Okay, this is my passport, but I haven't filled out the Health Declaration Form yet.

**检疫关员：**您现在可以填写纸质表格或通过微信小程序来填报。

Officer: You can do it now, either by filling out the paper form or through the WeChat app.

**旅客：**好的。我现在填写一下。

Passenger: OK. I'll fill it out now.

**检疫关员：**您在中国的联系电话没有填写。

Officer: You haven't filled in your telephone number in China.

**旅客：**好的。我现在就填写。是这样吗？

Passenger: I see. I'll fill it out right away. Is this right?

**检疫关员：**您这里填写的是境外的联系方式。请问您有境内的手机号码吗？

Officer: You've filled in your overseas contact information. Do you have a domestic mobile phone number?

**旅客：**有的。

Passenger: Yes, I do.

**检疫关员：**麻烦您修改一下。如果后续有需要的话，方便联系。

Officer: Please revise the information. This will make it convenient for us to contact you if necessary.

**检疫关员：**另外，您填写的航班号有误。麻烦修改后重新提交。

Officer: And the flight number that you've filled in is incorrect. Please fill in the right information and resubmit.

**旅客：**不好意思。我现在就修改。这样可以吗？

Passenger: I'm sorry. I'll do it right now. Is this okay?

**检疫关员：**可以。您还有其他需要申报的事项吗？

Officer: OK. Is there anything else you want to declare?

**旅客：**没有了，谢谢。

Passenger: Nothing else,thanks.

**检疫关员：**好的，因为您申报有一些症状，为了您和他人的健康，我们需要对您进行进一步的登记和检查。请随我到那边的房间。

Officer: Okay, because you indicate that you have some symptoms, we need to do some more registration and checking for your safety and that of others. Please come with me to the room over there.

**旅客：**好的，没问题。我完全配合。

Passenger: Sure, no problem. I'm totally okay with that.

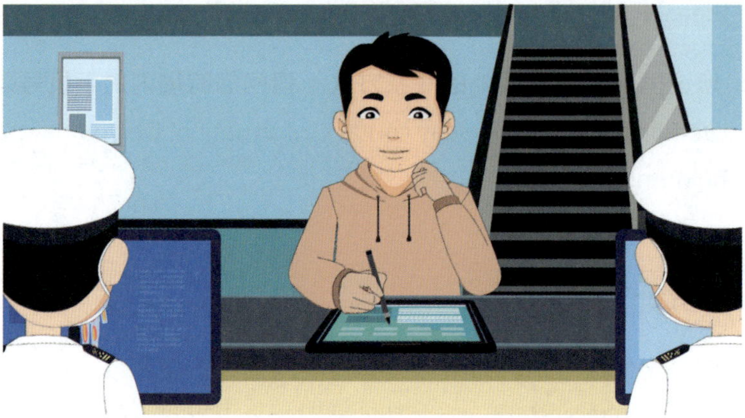

# 第二节 SECTION II 体温监测 TEMPERATURE MONITORING

## 场景一 体温正常

SCENE 1: NORMAL STATE

**检疫关员：** 旅客朋友们，前方是中国海关体温检测区域。请脱帽慢行。

Officer: Dear passengers, you're about to enter the temperature measuring area of China Customs. Please remove any headwear and slow down.

**检疫关员：** 抱小孩的旅客，请站在脚印处，将小孩的脸面向测温摄像头。

Officer: Passengers holding a child, please stand on the footprint sign, with your child facing the temperature camera.

**检疫关员：** 这位先生，麻烦您将帽子和墨镜摘下，准备测量体温。

Officer: Sir, please take off your hat and sunglasses and get ready for temperature measurement.

**检疫关员：** 这位女士，请让您的小孩一个接一个通过测温区域。

Officer: Madam, please let your children pass through the temperature measuring area one by one.

**检疫关员：**请排好队，保持一米间距，不要拥挤。

Officer: Please line up , keep a meter apart, and do not push.

## 场景二　体温复测

SCENE 2: TEMPERATURE REMEASUREMENT

**检疫关员：**先生，仪器显示您的体温高于正常值。请您退回黄线处重新测量。

Officer: Sir, the monitor shows your temperature is higher than normal. Please go back to the yellow line for remeasurement.

**（测温仪器再次报警）**

(The monitor alarms again)

**检疫关员：**请问您有哪里不舒服吗？

Officer: Do you feel any discomfort?

**旅客：**没有啊。我刚刚着急下飞机，可能穿多了热吧。

Passenger: No, I'm fine. I just got off the plane in a hurry, perhaps I dressed too warmly and I'm feeling overheated right now.

**检疫关员：**为了您和他人的健康，请随我到医学排查室。我们将用水银温度计为您复测体温。

Officer: For your safety and that of others, please come with me to the medical examination room. We'll take your temperature again using a mercury thermometer.

**旅客：**好的。

Passenger: Okay.

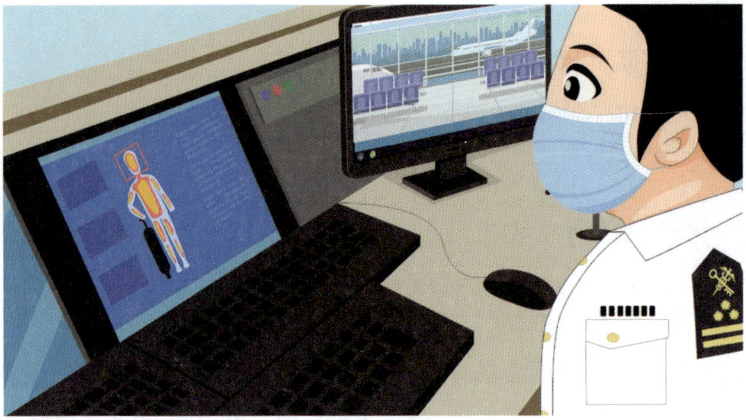

# 第三节 医学巡查

SECTION III MEDICAL INSPECTION

## 场景一 异常着装旅客

SCENE 1: PASSENGERS DRESSED UNTIMELY

**检疫关员：** 先生，您好，请问您是哪里不舒服吗？

Officer: Hello , sir, are you all right?

**旅客：** 是啊，我感觉很冷。

Passenger: Not really, I feel very cold.

**检疫关员：** 现在是 7 月份，大家都穿短袖呢，您怎么穿这么多？

Officer: It's July, and everyone wears short-sleeved clothes, but why do you dress so warm?

**旅客：** 上飞机前我感觉很热，上了飞机又觉得很冷，冷得发抖。

Passenger: It was hot before I boarded the plane, but as soon as I got on the plane, I was shivering with cold.

**检疫关员：**哦，这样啊。您从哪里过来的？这次旅行到过哪些国家或地区？

Officer: Oh, I see. Where did you come from? What countries or regions have you visited on this trip?

**旅客：**我是从马尼拉出发，经中国香港转机回来的。

Passenger: I set out from Manila and caught a connecting flight back home via Hong Kong, China.

**检疫关员：**就您一个人吗？还有没有同伴？

Officer: Are you traveling alone? Did you have a companion?

**旅客：**有个同伴和我一起到中国香港，不过他转机去别的地方了。

Passenger: I had a companion that flied with me to Hong Kong, China, but he had a connecting flight to somewhere else.

**检疫关员：**您或者您的同伴最近两周接触的人里有身体不舒服的吗？

Officer: Have you or your companion been in contact with anyone who feels unwell in the last two weeks?

**旅客：**有的，我同一个工地的好几个同事都住院了，医生说是疟疾。

Passenger: Yes, several of my coworkers on the same jobsite were hospitalized, and the doctor said it was malaria.

**检疫关员：**最近您有被蚊虫叮咬过吗？

Officer: Have you been bitten by mosquitoes recently?

**旅客：**每天都被咬。我们那儿蚊子太多了！

Passenger: Yes, I got bitten every day. We had too many mosquitoes there!

**检疫关员：**好的，根据您的描述，为了您和他人的健康，我们需要对您进行进一步的检查。请随我来。

Officer: All right, based on your description, and for your safety and that of others, we need to do some further exams. Please follow me.

**旅客：** 要做什么吗？

Passenger: What am I supposed to do?

**检疫关员：** 别担心，只是常规的信息登记和健康检查。

Officer: Don't worry, it's just a routine information registration and health checkup.

**旅客：** 那我的行李还没拿呢。

Passenger: But I haven't got my luggage yet.

**检疫关员：** 行李提取区还在前面。排查完如果无异常的话，您就可以去拿行李了。

Officer: The luggage claim area is down the hall. If everything turns out all right, you can go ahead and get your luggage.

**旅客：** 那好吧。

Passenger: Okay.

## 场景二 异常姿势旅客

SCENE 2: PASSENGERS IN UNUSUAL POSTURES

**检疫关员：** 您好，请问有什么需要帮助的吗？

Officer: Hello, what can I do for you?

**旅客：** 我妻子肚子疼。她需要坐在这里休息一下。

Passenger: My wife has a stomachache. She needs to sit down and have a rest.

**检疫关员：** 是哪里不舒服吗？

Officer: Is there something wrong?

**旅客：** 是啊，我们估计是吃坏了东西。从今天上飞机前就开始拉肚子，拉了有十几次。

Passenger: Yes, we probably ate some bad food. Before we got on the plane today, we began to have diarrhea and have used the bathroom a dozen times.

**旅客：** 你好，不好意思，我又想去上厕所。请问怎么走？

Passenger: Excuse me, I need to go to the bathroom again. Could you please tell me where the bathroom is?

**检疫关员：** 请随我来。我们有个专用的洗手间，请您上完厕所先别着急处理。我们需要您协助采集一点粪便样本，并对您进行进一步的排查和问诊。

Officer: Please follow me. We have a special bathroom, please do not exit the bathroom immediately after use. We need your assistance in taking a stool sample for further screening and testing.

**旅客：** 好的。

Passenger: Okay.

## 第四节 流行病学调查和医学排查

## SECTION IV EPIDEMIOLOGICAL INVESTIGATION AND MEDICAL SCREENING

### 场景一 疑似呼吸道传染病的流行病学调查和医学排查

### SCENE 1: EPIDEMIOLOGICAL INVESTIGATION AND MEDICAL SCREENING OF SUSPECTED CASES OF RESPIRATORY INFECTIOUS DISEASES

**检疫关员：** 请出示您的护照并告诉我以下信息：姓名、航班号、座位号、在华住址、联系电话、职业等。

Officer: Please show me your passport and provide the following information: personal name, flight number, seat number, address in China, phone number, occupation, etc.

**检疫关员：** 我们要给您测量一下体温。请把这支体温计夹在腋下 5 分钟。

Officer: We're going to take your temperature. Please keep this thermometer under your armpit for 5 minutes.

**检疫关员：** 您有没有感觉身体哪里不舒服？

Officer: How are you feeling?

**旅客：** 我有点累，可能坐太久飞机了。

Passenger: I'm a little tired, perhaps because of the long flight.

**检疫关员：** 您之前有量过体温吗？

Officer: Have you had your temperature taken before?

**旅客：** 就刚刚你们工作人员说我体温报警，但我在阿姆斯特丹机场那边也有测过，当时没有发烧。

Passenger: Just now, your colleague said that my temperature set the alarm off, but when I had my temperature taken at Amsterdam Airport, it didn't show that I had a fever at that time.

**检疫关员：** 那您最近 14 天有没有出现过什么症状，比如发热、咳嗽、呼吸困难、腹痛、腹泻等？

Officer: Have you experienced any symptoms, such as fever, cough, difficulty in breathing or stomachache in the last 14 days?

**旅客：** 3 天前有一点喉咙痛和流鼻涕。

Passenger: I had a sore throat and a runny nose 3 days ago.

**检疫关员：** 那有去看医生吗？有没有吃药？

Officer: Did you see a doctor or take any medicine?

**旅客：** 没有去看医生。我自己吃了两片奥司他韦就好了，现在没有什么症状。

Passenger: I haven't seen a doctor. I took two tablets of Oseltamivir and the symptoms are gone.

**检疫关员：** 14 天内您都到过哪些国家或地区？

Officer: Which countries or regions have you visited in the past 14 days?

**旅客：**美国和荷兰。我一周前从洛杉矶到阿姆斯特丹办事，昨天从阿姆斯特丹坐飞机来厦门。

Passenger: America and Holland. I travelled to Amsterdam from Los Angeles a week ago and flew to Xiamen from Amsterdam yesterday.

**检疫关员：**在 14 天内您是否接触过病人或疑似病人？

Officer: Have you ever been in contact with any confirmed or suspected patients in the past 14 days?

**旅客：**我应该没有接触过什么病人……哦，从洛杉矶出发前，也就是七八天前，我和一个表弟吃过晚饭，他患有感冒。

Passenger: No, I don't think so... Well, before I left Los Angeles seven or eight days ago, I had dinner with a cousin who had a cold.

**检疫关员：**您表弟感冒时有什么症状？他去医院了吗？现在好了吗？

Officer: What symptoms did your cousin have? Did he go to the hospital? Is he fine now?

**旅客：**他就是有点干咳吧，然后他自己也担心，前几天有去医院做过核酸检测。检测结果是阴性，但是我不知道他现在好了没。

Passenger: He just had a dry cough, but he was concerned and went to the hospital a few days ago for a nucleic acid test. The result was negative, but I don't know if he is all right now.

**检疫关员：**请把体温计取出。噢，体温是 38.6℃。

Officer: Please take out the thermometer. Oh, it's 38.6℃.

**旅客：**这么高啊，我还以为只是穿多了觉得热。

Passenger: It's so high, I thought it was just because I dressed too warm.

**检疫关员：**为了保护您和他人的身体健康，我需要对您采集样本进行检测，以排查传染病。

Officer: For your safety and that of others, I need to take a sample from you to check for any infectious disease.

**旅客：** 好的。

Passenger: Okay.

## 场景二 疑似消化道传染病的流行病学调查和医学排查

SCENE 2: EPIDEMIOLOGICAL INVESTIGATION AND MEDICAL SCREENING OF SUSPECTED CASES OF GASTROINTESTINAL INFECTIOUS DISEASES

**检疫关员：** 您好，请出示您的护照和登机牌。

Officer: Hello , please show me your passport and boarding pass.

**旅客：** 不好意思，我们的护照和登机牌在导游那里。

Passenger: Sorry, but our passports and boarding passes are with our tour guide.

**检疫关员：** 请联系你们的导游，让他也到这里来一下。

Officer: Please get your tour guide and ask him to come over here too.

**检疫关员：** 你们是跟团旅游吗？

Officer: Are you traveling with a tour group?

**旅客：** 是啊，女儿给我们报的旅游团。本来是想让我们放松一下，没想到又吐又拉的。

Passenger: Yes, our daughter signed us up for a tour. We just wanted to relax, but we didn't expect to suffer from diarrhea and vomiting.

**检疫关员：** 你们都有拉肚子和呕吐吗？还有没有其他的症状？

Officer: You both suffer from diarrhea and vomiting, right? Are there any other symptoms?

**旅客：** 我只是拉肚子，但是我妻子更严重。她还呕吐了好几次。

Passenger: I only have diarrhea, but my wife fares worse. She has also vomited several times.

**检疫关员：** 你们是什么时候开始出现症状的？

Officer: When did you start to have symptoms?

**旅客：** 我是今天早上开始拉肚子，我妻子也是差不多时间。她先是呕吐，然后开始拉肚子。

Passenger: I started to have diarrhea early this morning, and my wife began to have diarrhea around the same time. First, she vomited, and then she started to have diarrhea this morning.

**检疫关员：** 你们最近两周到过哪些国家或地区？能具体说说你们这几天的行程和吃了什么吗？

Officer: Which countries or regions have you visited in the last two weeks? And would you please tell me more about your trips and what you have eaten in the last few days?

**旅客：** 10 天前我们从厦门去泰国旅游。先是游览了曼谷，然后在清迈待了几天，之后去了芭提雅，昨天回到曼谷，今天回国。这几天都是吃的团餐，只有昨天晚上我们在街边夜市大排档吃了点海鲜，还喝了当地的特色水果饮料。我估计是食物不卫生，吃坏了肚子。

Passenger: We flied from Xiamen to Thailand 10 days ago. We toured Bangkok first, and then we stayed in Chiang Mai for a few days; afterwards, we went to Pattaya, and then we headed back to Bangkok yesterday, we're now back in China. All these days, we had meals with the group, but we had some seafood at a night-market food stall in the street last night, we also had local special fruit drinks. I think the food was not hygienic and, so we have diarrhea.

**检疫关员：** 今天你们在飞机上有吃东西吗？

Officer: Did you eat anything on the plane today?

**旅客：** 我们一点食欲也没有。在飞机上什么也没吃。

Passenger: We had no appetite at all. We didn't eat anything on the plane.

**（导游到场）**

(The tour guide arrives)

**检疫关员：**您是旅行团的跟团导游吗?

Officer: Are you the guide of the tour group?

**导游：**是的。

Tour Guide: Yes, I am.

**检疫关员：**这两位身体不舒服您知道吗?

Officer: Do you know that these two people are not feeling well?

**导游：**是的，我知道的。他们昨晚在路边的大排档吃东西吃坏了肚子，上吐下泻。

Tour Guide: Yes, I do. They ate something at a roadside food stall last night and suffer from vomiting and diarrhea.

**检疫关员：**好的，您既然知道您的团队中有人身体不舒服，就应该及时向机组工作人员报告。

Officer: Okay, since you know someone in your group is not feeling well, you should have notified the crew right away.

**导游：**对不起。是我疏忽了。我没想到他们的症状会变得这么严重。

Tour Guide: I'm sorry. I was negligent. I didn't expect their symptoms to become so serious.

**检疫关员：**你们旅行团里还有其他人有类似症状吗?

Officer: Does anyone else in your group have similar symptoms?

**导游：**没有，就他们两个昨晚脱离队伍自己行动。暂时没有听说其他人有不舒服的。

Tour Guide: No, they were the only two persons who went out last night. I haven't heard of anyone else who is feeling unwell.

**检疫关员：** 请您密切关注团员的身体健康情况，如果还有出现身体不适的，第一时间报告并及时上医院进行诊治。

Officer: Please pay close attention to the health condition of people in your group, and if there is anyone else who feels unwell, tell us right away and take him to the hospital for treatment without delay.

## 场景三 疑似蚊媒传染病的流行病学调查和医学排查

SCENE 3: EPIDEMIOLOGICAL INVESTIGATION AND MEDICAL SCREENING OF SUSPECTED CASES OF MOSQUITO-BORNE INFECTIOUS DISEASES

---

**检疫关员：** 您好，您发烧了，是吗？

Officer: Hello, you have a fever, right?

**旅客：** 是的，刚刚你们工作人员用体温计给我测了体温。

Passenger: Yes, your colleague has just taken my temperature with a mercury thermometer.

**检疫关员：** 您的健康申报卡上显示，您患有头痛、肌肉痛症状，最近还被蚊子叮咬过，是吗？

Officer: On the Health Declaration From, you indicate that you suffer from a headache and muscle pain, and you have got bitten by mosquitoes recently, right?

**旅客：** 是啊，蚊子太多了。

Passenger: Yes, there are just too many mosquitoes.

**检疫关员：** 我能看看您哪里被叮咬了吗？

Officer: Would you please show me where the mosquito bites are?

**旅客：** 胳膊、小腿，还有脖子这里。我已经被叮习惯了。

Passenger: On my arms and lower legs, and my neck as well. I've got used to being bitten by mosquitoes.

**检疫关员：** 嗯，我看您脖子和前胸这里有红色肿块。是平时就这样还是最近才出现的？

Officer: Well, I see red bumps on your neck and chest. Do you have them all the time or did they appear only recently?

**旅客：** 就这几天才这样，以前不会。

Passenger: They didn't appear until a couple of days ago.

**检疫关员：** 您最近一个月都去过哪些国家或地区？

Officer: Which countries or regions did you visit in the past month?

**旅客：** 我最近都在西哈努克市，在那儿待了半年多。

Passenger: I was in Sihanoukville for more than half a year.

**检疫关员：** 您在那里做什么？平时是住楼房还是平房？

Officer: What were you doing there? Did you live in an apartment building or a bungalow?

**旅客：** 我在那里做建筑工作。平时和工友们住在工地宿舍，那是一种临时搭建的平房。

Passenger: I was in a construction job there. I normally lived with my coworkers in the dormitory on the construction site, which was a makeshift bungalow.

**检疫关员：** 您的工友最近有生病的吗？

Officer: Has any of your coworkers been sick recently?

**旅客：** 是的，前几天有个工友去了医院，医生说他得了登革热。我不知道我是不是也得了登革热。

Passenger: Yes, a couple of days ago, a coworker went to the hospital, and the doctor said he had dengue fever. I don't know whether I have dengue fever or not.

**检疫关员：** 根据您描述的情况，我们不排除有蚊媒传染病的可能。我们需要对您采集一些血液样本进行后续的检测。

Officer: Based on your description, we can't rule out the possibility of a mosquito-borne disease. We need to take some blood samples from you for follow-up testing.

**旅客：** 这个检测要多少钱？

Passenger: How much will the test cost?

**检疫关员：** 检测是免费的。

Officer: The test is free.

**旅客：** 那太好了，帮我检测一下吧。

Passenger: Great, just do the test.

**检疫关员：** 请随我来。

Officer: Please come with me.

## 场景四 疑似其他传染病的流行病学调查和医学排查

SCENE 4: EPIDEMIOLOGICAL INVESTIGATION AND MEDICAL SCREENING OF SUSPECTED CASES OF OTHER INFECTIOUS DISEASES

**检疫关员：** 您好，您申报有淋巴结肿大和疾病接触史。能具体说说是什么情况吗？

Officer: Hello, you indicate that you have swollen lymph nodes and disease exposure. Would you please tell us what the situation is?

**旅客：** 你们这里的检查，信息是保密的吧？

Passenger: All information I give will be treated as confidential, right?

**检疫关员：** 请放心，您的所有信息都将被视为保密信息。

Officer: Please rest assured that all your information will be treated as confidential.

**旅客：** 您帮我看看。我脖子和耳朵后面这个是不是淋巴结肿大？有没有问题？

Passenger: Take a look. Do you see swollen lymph nodes in my neck and behind my ears? Are there any problems?

**检疫关员**：看起来是。您是什么时候发现的？还有没有其他不舒服的地方？

Officer: It looks like you do have a problem. When did you find them? Any other discomfort?

**旅客**：有半个月了。起初是发低烧，喉咙痛，然后就发现脖子、耳朵后面，甚至大腿根部都有小肿块。

Passenger: It's been half a month. At first, I had a low fever and a sore throat, and then I found small lumps in my neck, behind my ears, and even at the base of my thighs.

**检疫关员**：最近您有接触过什么病人吗？

Officer: Have you come into contact with any patients relatedly?

**旅客**：是这样的。半年前，我和朋友前往 T 国工作，在那里我曾经和陌生姑娘有过性接触。

Passenger: Here's the thing. Six months ago, my friend and I headed to Country T for work, I had sexual contact with a stranger girl there before.

**检疫关员**：您在当地看过医生吗？

Officer: Did you go to a doctor there?

**旅客**：我在那里没有医保，看病很贵，所以想这次回国检查一下。

Passenger: I didn't have health insurance there, and it was very expensive to see a doctor, so I want to have a check up this time back home.

**检疫关员**：我们可以采个血液样本进行艾滋病的快速筛查。

Officer: We can take a blood sample for a rapid HIV screening test.

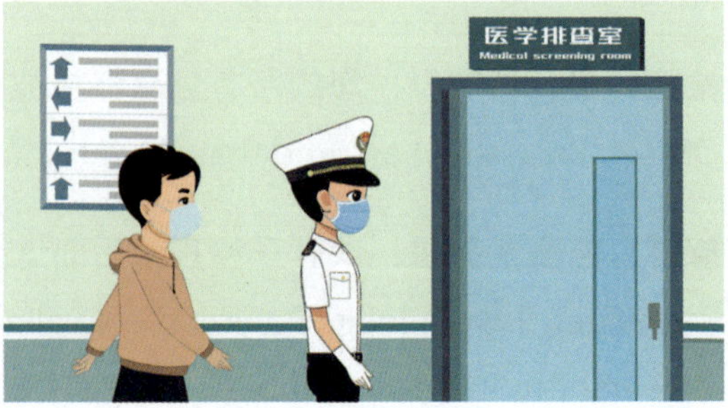


**旅客**：好的。

Passenger: Okay.

**（半小时后）**

(Half an hour later)

**检疫关员：** 快速筛查结果显示均为阴性。结合您目前症状，我们将转送您到医院进行进一步检查。请如实告知医生您近期的旅居史和接触史。

Officer: The rapid screening test turns out negative. Considering your current symptoms, we're going to transfer you to the hospital for further examination. Please be honest with the doctor about your recent history of travel and exposure.

**旅客：** 好的。

Passenger: Sure.

## 第五节 样本采集
## SECTION V SAMPLING

### 场景一 呼吸道样本采集
### SCENE 1: RESPIRATORY SAMPLING

**检疫关员：** 我们需要对您进行鼻咽拭子采集。这是采样知情同意书，请仔细阅读并签字。

Officer: We need to do a nasal throat swab test on you. This is the Informed Consent for Sampling, please read carefully and sign.

**检疫关员：** 这里有纸巾。如果在采样过程中您想打喷嚏，请用纸巾捂住口鼻。

Officer: Here are some tissues. If you sneeze during the sampling process, please cover your mouth and nose with tissues.

**检疫关员：** 您最近做过鼻腔手术吗？

Officer: Have you had a nasal surgery lately?

**旅客：** 没有。

Passenger: No , I haven't.

**检疫关员：**好的，我们先采集鼻拭子。这是一根棉签，薄而柔软。请放松，摘下口罩，仅露出鼻孔，把头后仰抬高，眼睛看天花板。保持住，好的，采好了。

Officer: Okay, we're going to take a nasal swab first. This is a cotton swab, thin and soft. Please relax, pull your mask down below your nose, tilt your head back and keep your eyes on the ceiling. Hold it that way, good, we're done.

**检疫关员：**接下来我们采集咽拭子。请张嘴。

Officer: Next, we're going to take a throat swab. Please open your mouth.

**旅客：**这样就好了吗?

Passenger: Is that good?

**检疫关员：**是的，请戴好口罩。

Officer: Yes, please put your mask back on.

**旅客：**请问多久我能知道检测结果?

Passenger: When can I get the test results?

**检疫关员：**检测结果会第一时间上传到便民服务线上平台，您可以通过您的手机移动客户端进行查看。

Officer: The test results will be uploaded to the Online Public Service Platform as soon as they become available, and you can check them through the app on your mobile phone.

## 场景二 血液样本采集

SCENE 2: BLOOD SAMPLING

**检疫关员：**现在我们要采集血液样本。请把袖子卷起来，胳膊放在桌面上。

Officer: Now we are going to take a blood sample. Please roll up your sleeves and put your arm on the table.

**旅客：** 我怕疼。能不能轻一点？

Passenger: I'm afraid it's going to hurt. I hope you can be a little gentler.

**检疫关员：** 请放心，不会疼的。

Officer: Please don't worry, it won't hurt.

**检疫关员：** 我们需要采集两管血液。请握紧拳头，放松拳头。摁住这里 5 分钟。不出血后，就可以将棉签丢到那边的医疗垃圾桶里。

Officer: We need to take two vials of blood. Please clench your fist, and release. Press here for 5 minutes. When the bleeding stops, throw the swab into the medical waste bin over there.

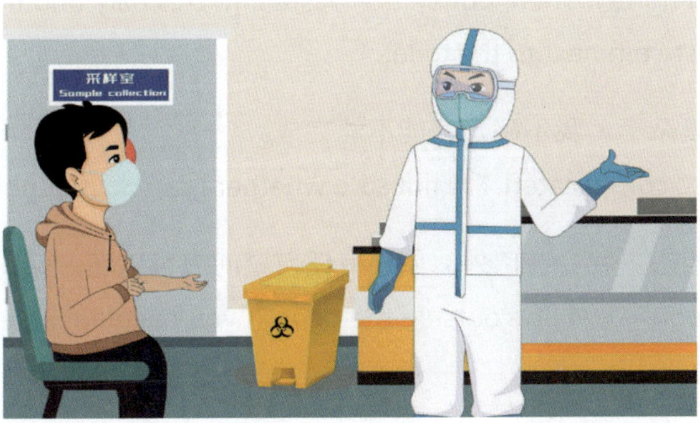


## 场景三 粪便样本采集

SCENE 3: STOOL SAMPLING

**检疫关员：** 我们需要对您进行粪便样本的采集。请问您现在想去洗手间吗？

Officer: We need to take a stool sample from you. Do you want to go to the bathroom now?

**旅客：** 是的，我肚子一直很不舒服。现在可以去了吗？

Passenger: Yes, my stomach has been feeling unwell all along. Can I go now?

**检疫关员：** 可以的，我们有一间专用洗手间，需要您配合我们采集一点粪便样品。

Officer: Sure, we have a special bathroom, and we need your help to take a stool sample.

**检疫关员：** 这里有一副手套、一根采样拭子、一个粪便采样杯和一个垃圾袋。排便后，请您戴好手套，用这根采样拭子取豌豆大小的粪便放入这个采样杯中，并拧紧盖子。然后将所有废物放入这个垃圾袋内，再丢到马桶旁边的医疗垃圾桶中。

Officer: Here are a pair of gloves, a sampling swab, a stool sampling cup and a waste bag. After bowel movements, please put on your gloves, use this sampling swab to take a pea-sized portion of the stool, put it into this sampling cup, and screw the lid on tightly. Then, put all the waste into this bag, and throw the bag in the medical waste bin next to the toilet.

**旅客：** 这个太复杂了。我不确定我能不能完成。

Passenger: It's so complicated. I'm not sure whether I can do it or not.

**检疫关员：** 别担心。我会在门外。如果有任何疑问您可以随时问我。

Officer: Don't worry. I will be outside the door. If you have any questions, you can ask me anytime.

**旅客：** 好吧，我试试看。

Passenger: Okay. I'll try my best.

## 第六节 转诊送医

## SECTION VI HOSPITAL TRANSFER

**检疫关员：** 根据您的症状、流行病学史和快速检测结果，我们需要将您转运至指定医院进一步诊治。

Officer: Based on your symptoms, epidemiological history and rapid test results, we need to transfer you to a designated hospital for further testing.

**旅客：** 可是我的妻子还在外面等我。我还要去找她。

Passenger: But my wife is still waiting for me outside. I have to get back to her.

**检疫关员：** 依照您目前的健康状况，您需要先去医院。您可以联系您的妻子先行办理通关手续。

Officer: Given your health status, you're required to go to the hospital first. You can ask your wife to go through Customs first.

**旅客：** 那我托运的行李怎么办？

Passenger: What about my checked luggage?

**检疫关员：** 您可以让您的妻子帮您提取行李，或者与航空公司工作人员协商将行李暂时寄放在机场。也可以由航空公司工作人员协助海关检查后交给您。

Officer: You can ask your wife to claim your luggage or talk to the airline staff and leave your luggage at the airport for the time being. Alternatively, the airline staff can assist the Customs to check your luggage and then hand it back to you.

**旅客：** 我要在医院住多久？

Passenger: How long will I have to stay in the hospital?

**检疫关员：** 那取决于您的健康状态和检测结果。具体的事项您可以咨询医院工作人员或当地卫生部门。

Officer: That depends on your health status and test results. For details,please consult the hospital staff or the local health department.

**旅客：** 那好吧，什么时候出发？

Passenger: All right，when do we set off?

**检疫关员：** 救护车马上就到。请您耐心等待。

Officer: The ambulance will arrive in a moment. Thank you for your patience.

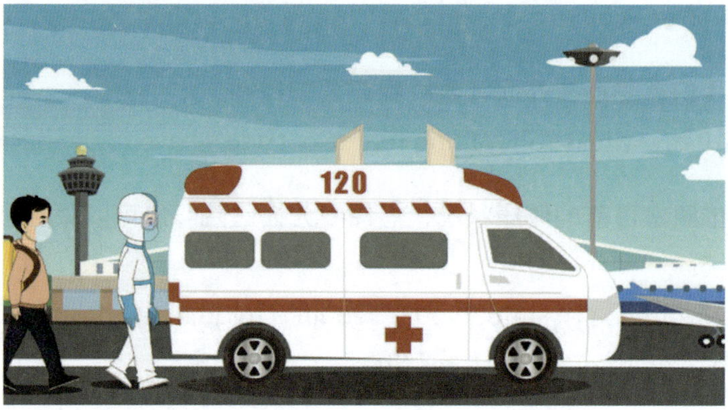


## 第七节 SECTION VII 卫生检疫人员相关表达 USEFUL EXPRESSIONS FOR QUARANTINE OFFICERS

1. 洗手间 / 行李提取区 / 边检手续柜台

Bathroom/Luggage Claim Area/Immigration Desk

2. 请往前走 / 左拐 / 右拐，您可以看到标志牌。

Please go straight ahead/turn left /turn right , and you will see the sign.

3. 请您佩戴好口罩。

Please wear a mask.

4. 请照顾好您的小孩并保管好您的随身物品。

Please do not leave your children unattended, and keep an eye on your belongings.

5. 请按一米间隔线有序排队。

Please line up and keep a meter apart.

6. 请出示您的护照 / 登机牌 / 采样二维码 / 病历 / 诊断报告 / 核酸检测报告。

Please show me your passport/boarding pass/sampling QR code/medical history/ diagnosis report/nucleic acid test report.

**7. 请将体温计夹在腋下 5 分钟，紧贴皮肤。**

Please keep the thermometer under your armpit for 5 minutes, press your arm against your body.

**8. 您接种过疫苗吗？**

Have you received any vaccinations?

**9. 您曾经感染过传染病吗？**

Have you ever contracted an infectious disease?

**10. 每个人都应该遵守海关的规章制度。**

Everyone should comply with Customs rules and regulations.

**11. 您的心情我们理解，但这是法律规定，希望您能理解并配合。**

We know how you feel, but this is a legal requirement and we hope you'll understand and cooperate.

**12. 请冷静。您这是妨碍海关关员执行正常工作任务。一切后果由您负责。**

Please calm down. You're interfering with the lawful duties of Customs officers. You'll be held responsible for all the consequences of your action.

# 第二章

CHAPTER II

# 入境交通工具卫生检疫

HEALTH QUARANTINE OF INBOUND VEHICLES

# 第一部分　航空器登临检疫

PART I　BOARDING AND QUARANTINE OF AIRCRAFT

## 第一节　一般流程

SECTION I　GENERAL PROCEDURES

**（地点：机舱门口）**

(Location: Cabin door)

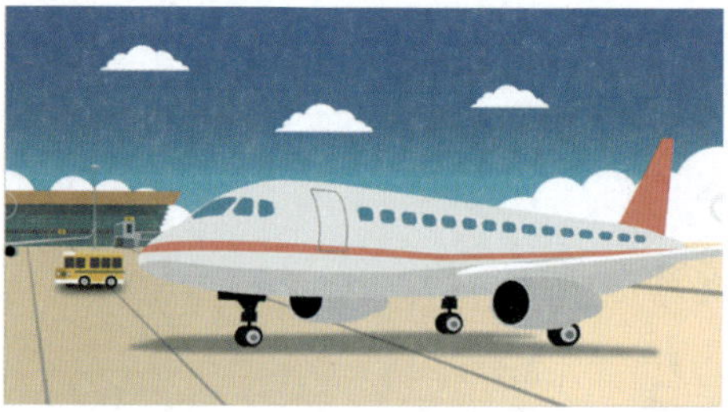

**检疫关员：**早上好，我们是中国海关关员。您是这架航班的乘务长吗？

Officer: Good morning, we're officers of China Customs. Are you the Chief Attendant for this flight?

**乘务长：**是的。早上好！

Chief Attendant: Yes, I am. Good morning!

**检疫关员：**欢迎来到厦门。乘务长，请您给我们简单介绍一下这趟航班的情况。我们需要跟总申报单核对。

Officer: Welcome to Xiamen. Chief Attendant, please give us a brief description of this flight. We'd like to verify the information on the General Declaration Form.

**乘务长：**没问题。这趟是新亚航空执飞，从巴厘岛直飞厦门的航班，航班号AB123，机号B123。航班于当地时间凌晨0点20分起飞，现在是北京时间5点40分。航程大约5个小时。机上有旅客236人，包括1位坐轮椅需要特殊陪护的旅客。机组总共11人，包括飞行员3人、乘务员7人、安全员1人。

Chief Attendant: No problem. This is a flight of New Asia Airlines from Bali to

Xiamen, with flight number AB123 and aircraft number B123. The flight took off at 0:20 am local time, and now it's 5:40 am Beijing time. The journey took about 5 hours. We have 236 passengers, including one wheelchaired passenger who requires special care. We have a crew of 11, including 3 pilots, 7 flight attendants and 1 safety officer.

**检疫关员：**236 名旅客……那飞机几乎坐满了吧？

Officer: 236 passengers... The flight is almost full, right?

**乘务长：**是的。巴厘岛—厦门是热门旅游航线，在这个假期，我们客座率基本上都能达到 90%。

Chief Attendant: Yes. The Bali-Xiamen route is a very popular flight route for tourists, and in this holiday period, we consistently have an occupancy rate of over 90%.

**检疫关员：**飞行过程还顺利吗？

Officer: Did the flight go smoothly?

**乘务长：**谢谢您的关心。除了有一次气流颠簸，飞行过程中一切顺利。

Chief Attendant: Thanks for your concern. We had a rather smooth flight, except for a brief turbulence encounter.

**检疫关员：**机组成员感觉怎么样？有没有身体不舒服的？

Officer: How do the crew feel? Does anyone feel unwell?

**乘务长：**有些累。您知道的，我们这条航线是安排在午夜后起飞，旅客又比较多。这确实会比较辛苦一些，但是我们感觉还好。

Chief Attendant: We're a little tired. You know, the flight was scheduled for take-off after midnight, and with so many passengers. It was indeed a tough flight, but we feel fine.

**检疫关员：**晚间工作确实辛苦。有没有旅客感到身体不舒服的？或者您有没有注意到不寻常的旅客，如发烧、咳嗽、恶心、呕吐、腹泻、皮疹、黄疸？

Officer: Working at night is really hard. Have any passengers complained of any discomfort? Or have you noticed any passengers with a fever, cough, nausea, vomiting, diarrhea, rash or jaundice?

**乘务长：** 我想想……应该都没有。

Chief Attendant: Let me see... None, I think.

**检疫关员：** 有没有发现飞机上有蚊子、苍蝇、老鼠、蟑螂出没，特别是配餐间、洗手间这些地方？

Officer: Have you seen any mosquitoes, flies, rodents or cockroaches on the plane, especially in the galley and restrooms?

**乘务长：** 没有发现老鼠、虫子之类的。我们非常重视环境卫生。

Chief Attendant: We haven't seen any rodents or insects. We take environmental hygiene very seriously.

**检疫关员：** 好的。您看下这张总申报单，这里的健康部分是空白的。

Officer: All right. Take a look at this General Declaration Form, the Declaration of Health is blank.

**乘务长：** 我去过很多航空口岸，但是他们都没要求我填写这部分。这是额外的要求吗？

Chief Attendant: I've been to many airports, but I've never been asked to fill in this part. Is this an extra requirement?

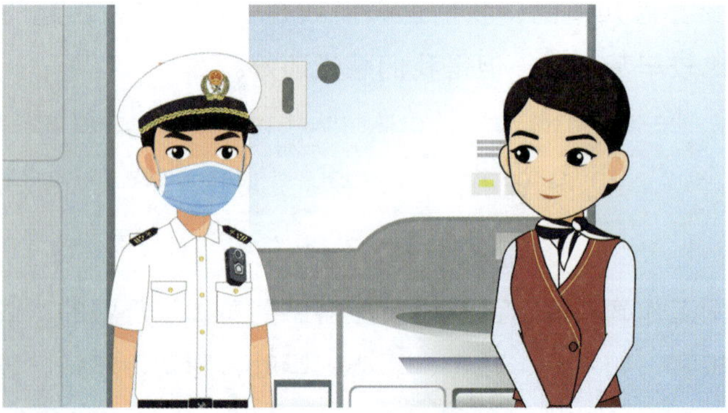

**检疫关员**：总申报单上相关信息必须填写清楚并且由机长签字。这不仅是中国的卫生检疫法规的要求，也是《国际卫生条例》的规定。

Officer: All information required on the General Declaration Form must be filled in clearly, and the form must be signed by the Captain. This is not only a requirement of Chinese health and quarantine laws, but also a stipulation in the *International Health Regulations.*

**乘务长**：明白了。那我现在填写完拿给机长签字后给您。

Chief Attendant: I see. I'll fill it in right away and have it signed by the Captain, here you are.

**检疫关员**：申报信息核对无误，我们现在要对本航班进行现场检查，请您和其他机组成员配合我们。在海关检查完成之前，未经海关允许，任何人不得上下飞机，不准装卸行李、货物、邮包等物品。

Officer: We've verified the information on the Declaration Form, and we're now going to inspect the flight, we expect you and your fellow crew members to cooperate with us. Before our inspection is completed and without our permission, no one is allowed to get on or off the plane, and no luggage, cargo, parcels or other items can be moved.

**乘务长**：好的。我们会全力配合。

Chief Attendant: Okay. We'll fully cooperate with you on all this.

**检疫关员**：开始检查之前，我们要先对旅客进行广播告知。

Officer: Before the inspection, we would like to make an announcement to the passengers.

**乘务长**：好的。您可以用机上的广播系统。我带您过去。

Chief Attendant: Sure. You can use the passenger address system onboard. Please follow me.

**检疫关员**：（广播）各位旅客，你们好，欢迎来到厦门。我们是中国海关关员，现在我们要在机上进行检查。请所有旅客全部坐于原位，不要起身走动或者拿取行李，保持通道畅通。感谢您的配合！

Officer: (Passenger announcement) Dear passengers, welcome to Xiamen. We're officers of China Customs, and we're going to inspect this aircraft. Please remain seated and do not stand up or move your luggage, and please keep the aisle clear. Thank you for your cooperation!

**（机上巡查）**

(Cabin inspection)

**检疫关员：**乘务长，有一些旅客的行李堵住了过道，请让旅客把行李挪开，方便工作人员通过。

Officer: Chief Attendant, the aisle is blocked by some luggage. Please ask the passengers to remove it so that we can walk through.

**乘务长：**好的。

Chief Attendant: Sure.

**检疫关员：**（询问另一名乘务员）有旅客或机组成员感到身体不舒服的吗？有发现蚊子、苍蝇、蟑螂或者老鼠之类的吗？

Officer: (To a flight attendant) Did any passenger or crew member complain of any discomfort? And did you see any mosquitoes, flies, cockroaches or rodents?

**乘务员：**据我所知都没有。

Attendant: Not that I know of.

**检疫关员：**有发现什么需要申报的异常情况吗？

Officer: Did you notice anything unusual that you need to declare?

**乘务员：**也没有。

Attendant: Nope.

**检疫关员：**（对机长说）一切正常。请您在海关进出境运输工具登临检查记录单上签字。

Officer: (Tell the captain) Everything is all right. Please sign this Customs Onboard

Inspection Record of Inbound and Outbound Conveyance.

**机长：**好的。

Captain: Okay.

**检疫关员：**感谢您的配合。海关的登临检疫到此结束。您可以安排人员上下飞机和卸货了。

Officer: Thank you for your cooperation. This is the end of Customs quarantine. People are now allowed to get on or off the plane and load or unload goods.

**乘务长：**谢谢！

Chief Attendant: Thank you very much!

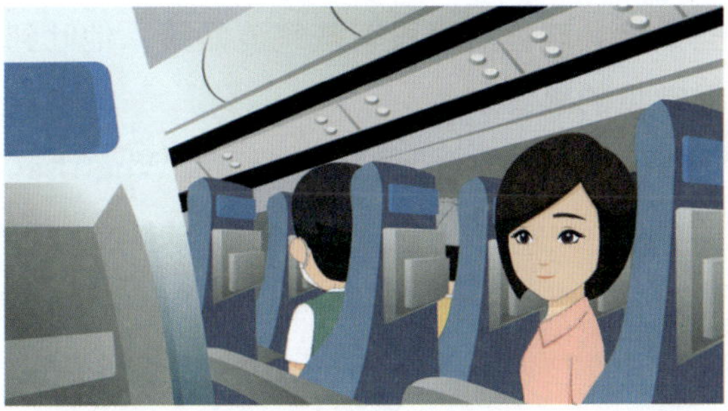

## 第二节 机上巡查
## SECTION II INSPECTION ONBOARD

### 场景一 航空器运营方申报有晕机症状旅客
### SCENE 1: DECLARATION OF THE AIRCRAFT OPERATOR CONCERNING A PASSENGER WITH AIRSICKNESS SYMPTOMS

**（地点：机舱门口）**

(Location: Cabin door)

**检疫关员：** 您好！有没有旅客感到身体不舒服的？或者您有没有注意到不寻常的旅客，如发烧、咳嗽、恶心、呕吐、腹泻、皮疹、黄疸？

Officer: Hello! Have any passengers complained of any discomfort? Or have you noticed any passengers with fever, cough, nausea, vomiting, diarrhea, rash or jaundice?

**乘务长：** 是有一个旅客不太舒服。

Chief Attendant: One of the passengers doesn't feel well.

**检疫关员：** 具体是什么情况呢？

Officer: What has happened?

**乘务长：** 是一名来自新加坡的旅客。送餐的时候我们看他脸色不太好。他说他昨晚没休息好，又有些晕机。航程后半段有些气流颠簸，他吐到了袋子里。情况不是很严重。晕机是很常见的事。

Chief Attendant: It's a passenger from Singapore. When serving the meal, we noticed that he didn't look very well. He said he didn't sleep well last night and felt airsick. The flight encountered turbulence during its second half, and he vomited into the bag. It wasn't a very serious situation. Airsickness is a rather common occurrence.

**检疫关员：** 好的，你们有采取什么处理措施吗？

Officer: Well, did you take any measures?

**乘务长：** 我们本来想给他调换到最后一排单独坐，但是今天航班已经客满，后排几乎没有空位。加上旅客一直坚持说没有大碍，我们就给他提供了一些晕机药和温水。

Chief Attendant: We could have put him in the last row, so that he could sit alone, but the flight today is quite full and almost all the back-row seats are occupied. And the passenger insists that he's fine, so we've just handed him some airsickness pills and hot water.

**检疫关员：** 这名旅客坐在哪里？

Officer: Where is the passenger seated?

**乘务长：**他坐在前舱第 41 排左边靠过道位置。

Chief Attendant: He's in an aisle seat in the 41st row, on the left side.

**检疫关员：**您能带我去看看他的情况吗？

Officer: Can we check on the passenger?

**乘务长：**好的。这边走。

Chief Attendant: Sure. This way please.

**（走到旅客座位跟前）**

(Walking up to the passenger)

**检疫关员：**您好，我们是海关关员。您现在感觉怎么样？

Officer: Hello, we're Customs Officers. How do you feel now?

**旅客：**好多了。有一阵飞机颠簸得厉害，我感觉恶心就吐了，现在舒服多了。

Passenger: Much better now. The flight was very bumpy a while ago, and I felt nauseous and vomited, but I feel much better now.

**检疫关员：**以前也会这样吗？平时会晕机或者晕车吗？

Officer: Did you have similar experiences in the past? Do you usually get airsick or carsick?

**旅客：**一直都会。每次上飞机耳朵就嗡嗡嗡地响，胃里翻江倒海的。特别难受，这次也不例外。

Passenger: I always do. Whenever I'm on a plane, I hear a ringing in my ears and my stomach churns. It's awful, and this flight is no exception.

**检疫关员：**吐的是什么东西？

Officer: What's in your vomit?

**旅客：**是我的晚饭，有米饭、青菜、鸡蛋等。

Passenger: My dinner—rice, vegetables, eggs, etc.

**检疫关员：** 在飞机上有吃东西吗？

Officer: Did you eat anything during the flight?

**旅客：** 没有。我一点食欲也没有。

Passenger: No. I had no appetite at all.

**检疫关员：** 请问您是从哪里上的飞机？又去过哪些城市？

Officer: Where did you board this plane? And which cities have you visited?

**旅客：** 我是在新加坡上的飞机。之前一直在我位于新加坡的家里。

Passenger: I got on the plane in Singapore. Before that, I stayed at home in Singapore.

**检疫关员：** 您今天早、午、晚餐吃的是什么？能回忆起来吗？

Officer: What did you have for breakfast, lunch and dinner today? Do you still remember them?

**旅客：** 没什么特别的。我的晚餐是父母亲在家里准备的，有白米饭、青菜和炒鸡蛋。午餐吃的肯德基的鸡腿堡和可乐，早餐吃的牛奶和面包。

Passenger: Nothing special. My dinner had been prepared by my parents at home, and it was steamed rice, green vegetables and a scrambled egg. I had a KFC zinger burger and coke for lunch, and milk and bread for breakfast.

**检疫关员：** 除了呕吐之外，还有其他不舒服的吗？比如肚子痛、拉肚子、头晕、胸闷、喘不上气之类的？

Officer: Do you feel any discomfort other than vomiting, such as stomachache, diarrhea, dizziness, chest tightness and shortness of breath?

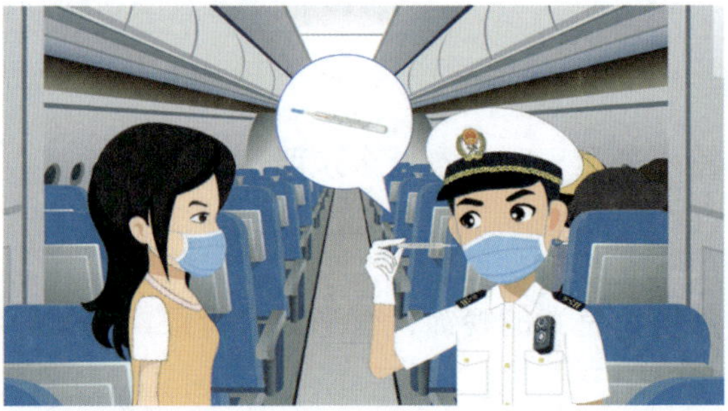

**旅客：** 都没有。

Passenger: Nope.

**检疫关员：**我们需要给您测个体温。

Officer: We need to take your temperature.

**旅客：**好的。

Passenger: Okay.

**检疫关员：**（测量体温）体温 36.5℃。谢谢您的配合。如果下机后还有不舒服，一定要去看医生，同时告诉医生您近期的旅行情况。

Officer: (Measuring the passenger's temperature) It's 36.5℃. Thank you for your cooperation. If you still feel unwell after getting off, go see a doctor and tell him about your recent travel history.

**旅客：**好的，谢谢您的提醒。我现在感觉非常好。

Passenger: All right. Thanks a lot. I feel pretty good now.

**检疫关员：**（对乘务长说）看起来只是晕机。本次航班所有旅客可以按照正常流程下机。

Officer: (Tell the Chief Attendant)Seems it is just a case of airsickness. All passengers on this flight can get off according to the normal procedure.

**乘务长：**好的，谢谢！

Chief Attendant: Great, thank you very much!

## 场景二 航空器运营方申报有发热及呼吸道症状旅客

SCENE 2: DECLARATION OF THE AIRCRAFT OPERATOR CONCERNING A PASSENGER WITH FEVER AND RESPIRATORY SYMPTOMS

**（背景：15 分钟前，海关接到机场指挥中心报告来自 P 国的 AB123 号航班上有 1 名旅客出现发热症状）**

(Background: 15 minutes ago, the Customs received a report from the airport command center that a passenger on Flight AB123 from Country P had fever symptoms)

**（地点：机舱门口）**

(Location: Cabin door)

**检疫关员：**您好，乘务长，是您向地面中心报告有一名旅客发热吗？

Officer: Hello, Chief Attendant, did you report to the ground center that one of the passengers has a fever?

**乘务长：**是的。当发现任何旅客发烧时，我们必须向目的地海关申报。是这样吧？

Chief Attendant: Yes. We're required to declare to the Customs at the destination, when any passenger is found to have a fever. Is that so?

**检疫关员：**是的，您做得很好。请告诉我们是什么情况。

Officer: Yes. You've done a great job. Please tell us what has happened.

**乘务长：**是这样的。登机前，我们测量了所有旅客的体温，一切都很正常。飞行途中，乘务员注意到有位旅客脸色发红，呼吸急促。她用体温计给他测温，显示38.2℃。因此，我们立即向地面部门报告。

Chief Attendant: Well. Before boarding, we took the temperature of all the passengers and everything was fine. During the flight, an attendant noticed that one of the passengers looked flushed and was short of breath. She measured his temperature with a thermometer, and it was 38.2℃. So,we immediately reported it to the ground center.

**检疫关员：**你们测体温用的是什么设备？

Officer: What kind of thermometer did you use?

**乘务长：**额温枪。应该是准确的，因为我们定期会校准。

Chief Attendant: A forehead thermometer. It should be accurate, because we calibrate it regularly.

**检疫关员：**还有什么要报告的吗？

Officer: Is there anything else to be reported?

**乘务长：**没有了，其他一切正常。

Chief Attendant: No,everything is fine.

**检疫关员：**好的。你们有做什么临时处置吗？

Officer: Good. Did you take any temporary measures?

**乘务长：**我们把那名旅客调换到了远离其他乘客的最后一排预留座位，并提供了一次性口罩和手套。

Chief Attendant: We moved the passenger to a reserved seat in the last row, far away from other passengers, and we handed him a disposable mask and gloves.

**检疫关员：**处理得不错。带我去看看情况。你们有询问过旅客什么时候开始不舒服吗？

Officer: Good job. Take me to the passenger. Did you ask him when he started feeling unwell?

**乘务长：**有的。这名旅客说他最近一周都有些感冒咳嗽，前一晚还发烧了。上飞机前吃了退烧药感觉好一些了。

Chief Attendant: Yes. The passenger said he had a cold and coughed a lot last week, and he had a fever the night before. He felt better after taking some antipyretics before boarding the plane.

**检疫关员：**他有去过洗手间吗？是哪一间？

Officer: Did he use the restroom? Which one did he use?

**乘务长：**是后舱靠左边的那一间。

Chief Attendant: The one on the left side of the rear cabin.

**检疫关员：**哪些乘务员为这名旅客提供过服务？

Officer: Which flight attendants served this sick passenger?

**乘务长：**乘务员 A 和 B。

Chief Attendant: Flight attendants A and B.

**检疫关员：** 先生，您好，您还好吗？

Officer: Hello , sir, are you all right?

**旅客：** 咳嗽……嗯，还有头痛。

Passenger: I have a cough... um, and a headache.

**检疫关员：** 让我们为您测量一下腋温。请把水银温度计夹在腋下 5 分钟。

Officer: We're going to take your armpit temperature. Please keep this thermometer under your armpit for five minutes.

**检疫关员：** 您是什么时候开始出现症状的呢？

Officer: When did you get the symptoms?

**旅客：** 我想想…… 我是一周前开始咳嗽，3 天前开始头痛。

Passenger: Let me see... I started coughing a week ago and had a headache three days ago.

**检疫关员：** 您去医院就诊过吗？

Officer: Did you go to a doctor?

**旅客：** 去过了。医生说我感冒了，给我开了一些感冒药。

Passenger: Yes, I did. The doctor said I had a cold and gave me some pills for my cold.

**检疫关员：** 您吃了药之后有好转吗？

Officer: Did you get better after taking the pills?

**旅客：** 有的。之前我的体温是 38.6℃，现在已经降下来一些了。

Passenger: Yes. My body temperature was 38.6℃, but it has dropped a little bit.

**检疫关员：** 请您把体温计拿出来给我。

Officer: Please take out the thermometer.

**（递体温计）**

(Thermometer handed to the Officer)

**检疫关员：** 让我看看……现在是 38.3℃。

Officer: Let me have a look... It's 38.3℃.

**旅客：** 又发烧了。难怪我头痛。

Passenger: I have a fever again. No wonder my head hurts.

**（安排同行人员）**

(Making arrangements for fellow travelers)

**检疫关员：** 这位旅客原本的座位在哪里？他前后三排和同一排旅客，以及给他提供过服务的空乘人员都视为密切接触者。其他旅客可以先下飞机，然后是密切接触者。旅客本人最后一个离开飞机。

Officer: Where was this passenger seated in the beginning? The passengers in the three rows around him and those in the same row as him, as well as the flight attendants who have served him, are close contacts. Other passengers can get off the plane first, followed by the close contacts. The sick passenger will be the last one to go.

**乘务长：** 好的。我们会配合做好安排。

Chief Attendant: All right. We'll fully cooperate with you on all this.

**检疫关员：** 由于飞机上发现传染病疑似病例，按规定飞机需要实施终末消毒，我们会在现场进行全程监督。请在所有人员都下飞机之后通知我们前来监管终末消毒。

Officer: Since a suspected case of infection has been found, the plane must undergo terminal disinfection as required. We'll supervise the terminal disinfection on the spot from start to finish. Please notify us after all people get off, and we'll come back to supervise the terminal disinfection.

**乘务长：** 好的。我现在通知地面人员安排消毒人员过来。

Chief Attendant: Okay. I'll ask the ground personnel to send disinfection workers over.

## 场景三 机上巡查发现有消化道症状旅客

SCENE 3: DETECTION OF A PASSENGER WITH GASTROINTESTINAL INFECTION SYMPTOMS DURING ONBOARD INSPECTION

**（机上巡查）**

(Onboard inspection)

**检疫关员（小王）：**小张，您看那边那位旅客捂着肚子坐立不安的，是不是不太舒服？

Officer (Xiao Wang): Xiao Zhang, look at the passenger over there, the one who looks agitated, with his hands on his stomach. He seems to be in pain, doesn't he?

**检疫关员（小张）：**看起来确实是。我去问一下。您也跟乘务长了解一下情况。

Officer (Xiao Zhang): It looks like so. I'll go check it out. You may talk to the Chief Attendant for more detail.

**检疫关员（小王）：**好的。

Officer (Xiao Wang): Okay.

**检疫关员（小王）：**乘务长，那边有位旅客看起来不太舒服。你们之前有注意到她有什么异常吗？

Officer (Xiao Wang): Chief Attendant, it seems that a passenger over there doesn't feel well. Did you notice anything abnormal about her?

**乘务长：**噢！那位女士啊，她刚才吐了，我们才请她去后排就座的。

Chief Attendant: Oh! That lady, she vomited a while ago, so we moved her to a seat in the back row.

**检疫关员（小王）：**具体是什么情况？

Officer (Xiao Wang): What has happened?

**乘务长：**她是一名来自英国跟团旅游的旅客。飞行途中吐了两三次，弄脏了座椅和地板。我们给她调换了座位。她中间还去了几趟洗手间，可能还拉肚子了。

Chief Attendant: She is from Britain and is a member of a tour group. She vomited two or three times during the flight, staining the seat and the floor. We moved her to another seat. She also made several trips to the restroom, maybe she's got diarrhea.

**检疫关员（小王）：**她有同行人员吗？

Officer (Xiao Wang): Does she have any companion?

**乘务长：**她的丈夫和她一起，也是英国人，跟她坐同一排。他看起来没什么异常。

Chief Attendant: Her husband is with her, he is also British and sits in the same row as her. He looks fine, though.

**检疫关员（小王）：**你们做了什么处理呢？

Officer (Xiao Wang): What have you done with her?

**乘务长：**我们请她到后排座位单独就坐，和其他旅客分开，并且将后舱厕所给她单独使用。有专门的乘务人员为她提供服务。

Chief Attendant: We moved her to the back row, where she could sit alone away from other passengers, and the lavatory in the rear cabin was reserved for her. One of our attendants was assigned to serve her.

**检疫关员（小王）：**做得很好。呕吐物是怎么处理的？

Officer (Xiao Wang): Good job. How did you deal with the vomit?

**乘务长：**乘务人员拿湿巾清理了地面和座椅上的呕吐物，然后将它们扔到了洗手间的垃圾桶里。

Chief Attendant: An attendant cleaned the vomit from the floor and the seat using wet tissues, and then threw them into the waste bin in the restroom.

**检疫关员（小王）：** 直接扔掉还不行。这些呕吐物都需要消毒。机上有配备消毒剂吗？

Officer (Xiao Wang): That's not enough. The vomit must be disinfected. Do you have any disinfectant on the plane?

**乘务长：** 有消毒片。我马上安排人去消毒。

Chief Attendant: We have disinfection tablets. I'll send someone to disinfect the vomit right away.

**检疫关员（小王）：** 乘务人员有做个人防护吗？

Officer (Xiao Wang): Did the attendants have proper personal protection?

**乘务长：** 引导她和给她提供服务的乘务员都戴了手套和一次性口罩。处理呕吐物的乘务员还戴了橡胶手套。没有其他人与她有过直接接触。

Chief Attendant: The attendants who guided her and who served her wore gloves and disposable masks. The attendant who dealt with the vomit wore rubber gloves. No one else has had direct contact with her.

**检疫关员（小王）：** 处理得非常专业。有意识地让她尽量减少与其他人员的密切接触和不必要的接触，看得出来你们应对这种情况很有经验。

Officer (Xiao Wang): You've been very professional. I can tell that you're very experienced in dealing with such situations, taking great care to prevent her from having close contact and unnecessary contact with others.

**乘务长：** 谢谢。我们公司有应对这种情况的标准操作规程，乘务组也都进行过培训。

Chief Attendant: Thanks. My company has standard operating procedures for dealing with such situations, and the crew have also been trained.

**检疫关员（小王）：** 不错，不过还可以做得更好。遇到这种情况，除了要做好规范的机上紧急处置，还应该及时向地面中心报告并且向海关申报。此外，总申报单的卫生部分也要做好记录。

Officer (Xiao Wang): Not bad, but you could have done better. Under such circumstances, you should not only follow the standard onboard emergency response procedures, but also promptly inform the ground center and declare to the Customs. Besides, you should record the information in the Declaration of Health on the General Declaration Form.

**乘务长：** 明白了。下次碰到有类似的情况我们一定及时报告。
Chief Attendant: All right. We'll immediately inform the ground center when we're caught in a similar situation again.

**检疫关员（小王）：** 还有一件事，机上被呕吐物或者呼吸道分泌物、血液、腹泻物等污染的客舱区域都要及时消毒。不要用手直接接触污染物，最好是用吸附性消毒剂消毒，再用拾取铲之类的工具将凝固的污染物铲入专用的生物危害垃圾袋，处理后要做好手的消毒。这样有助于保护你们和其他乘客的安全。
Officer (Xiao Wang): One more thing, any part of the cabin contaminated by vomit, respiratory secretions, blood or diarrhea must be disinfected immediately. Do not touch the contaminants with your hands. Adsorbent disinfectant is preferred. Congealed contaminants must be scraped up with a proper tool, such as a scoop, and then placed into a special biohazard waste bag. After everything is done, be sure to disinfect your hands. This will help keep you and other passengers safe.

**乘务长：** 谢谢您的提醒。我们也会向公司建议把这点写进我们的标准处置流程。
Chief Attendant: Thank you for the information. We'll also suggest to our company to include this in our standard response procedures.

**检疫关员（小张）：** 小王，刚刚问了一下情况。那位女士是英国人，最近一周在跟团旅游。上个星期他们去了 M 国、T 国、P 国，接下来一周打算在厦门旅游。昨天晚上在 P 国，她和她丈夫在路边摊吃了海鲜烧烤、三文鱼芒果沙拉、凉拌青木瓜，还喝了奶茶。今天早上早些时候，她觉得肚子痛、头痛、恶心，上吐下泻，在飞机上吐了两次，腹泻两次都是水样便。给她量了体温，37.2℃。
Officer (Xiao Zhang): Xiao Wang, I've just asked some questions. She is from Britain and has joined a tour group for a week. They visited Country M, Country T, and Country P last week, and they're going to tour Xiamen next week. Last night in

the Country P, she and her husband had seafood barbecues, salmon mixed with mango salads, and green papaya salads at roadside stalls, and they also drank milk tea. Earlier this morning, she had a stomachache and a headache and felt nauseous, and she then vomited and had loose bowels. She vomited twice and passed loose, watery stool twice on the flight. Her body temperature was checked, and it was 37.2℃.

**检疫关员（小王）：**她丈夫有不舒服吗？

Officer (Xiao Wang): Is her husband okay?

**检疫关员（小张）：**据她说，她丈夫昨天半夜也腹泻了两次，但是今天症状消失了。

Officer (Xiao Zhang): She said that her husband also had loose bowels twice late last night , but the symptom has gone away today.

**检疫关员（小王）：**乘务长，这对夫妇需要接受医学检查。您先安排其他旅客和机组成员分批按顺序下飞机。这对夫妇在后排等待，最后再下。

Officer (Xiao Wang): Chief Attendant, the couple need to undergo medical screenings. You may let the other passengers and the crew get off in groups. The couple will be waiting in the back row, and they will be the last two passengers to leave.

**乘务长：**好的，我去通知地面人员和乘务组安排旅客下飞机。

Chief Attendant: Okay, I'll ask the ground staff and the crew to arrange for the passengers to get off.

**检疫关员（小王）：**这对夫妇还有没有同行人员？让我看一下乘客名单。

Officer (Xiao Wang): Does the couple have any companions? Let me take a look at the passenger list.

**乘务长：**我让人去拿。还有什么需要我们做的吗？

Chief Attendant: I'll send someone to get the list. What else can we do?

**检疫关员（小王）：**由于机上发现有消化道症状的疑似病例，飞机必须进行终末消毒。我们会给您开具检验检疫处理通知书。

Officer (Xiao Wang): Since there're suspected cases of gastrointestinal infection onboard, the plane must undergo terminal disinfection. We'll issue a Notification of Inspection and Quarantine Treatment to you.

**乘务长：**好的。我马上打电话联系地面部门，他们会让检疫处理公司派人过来。

Chief Attendant: All right. I'll call contact the ground department right away, and they'll ask the quarantine treatment company to send someone over.

**（旅客、机组下机）**

(Passengers and crew disembarking)

**[检疫关员（小张）护送有症状旅客离开]**

(Symptomatic passengers escorted off the plane by Officer Xiao Zhang )

**乘务长：**这些消毒剂对人体有害吗？我有些担心。喷洒后的残留物是否会一直残留在机舱里散发毒性，或者损坏飞机上的设备？

Chief Attendant: Is this disinfectant harmful to humans? I'm a little concerned. After spraying, will it the residues remain in the cabin cockpit and release toxic substances or damage the equipment on the plane?

**检疫关员（小王）：**别担心。我们要求使用的消毒剂都是经民航主管部门批准可以在飞机上使用的。

Officer (Xiao Wang): Don't worry. All the disinfectants we require have been appr-oved by civil aviation authorities for use on aircraft.

**乘务长：**好的。

Chief Attendant: All right.

**[检疫关员（小王）检查消毒剂的颜色，并做了记录]**

(Officer Xiao Wang checks the color of the disinfectant and makes a record)

**检疫关员（小王）：**请关闭飞机出口和舱门，将通风量调至最大，使客舱进行一次完整换气。

Officer (Xiao Wang): Please close the exit and cabin doors of the plane, and turn the ventilator up to the maximum to give the cabin a complete air change.

**乘务长：** 好的。

Chief Attendant: Okay.

**检疫关员（小王）：** 现在可以开始消毒了。消毒作业时请关闭空调系统。

Officer (Xiao Wang): You can start the disinfection now. Please keep the air-conditioning system off during the disinfection.

**乘务长：** 好的。空调系统都已经关闭。

Chief Attendant: Okay. The air-conditioning system is off.

**检疫关员（小王）：** 请您打开所有行李架和卫生间门，所有机组成员在地面等候消毒完成。

Officer (Xiao Wang): Please open all the overhead storage compartments and lavatory doors, and the crew shall wait on the ground until the disinfection is completed.

**乘务长：** 所有机组成员吗？

Chief Attendant: All the crew?

**检疫关员（小王）：** 是的，包括机长。

Officer (Xiao Wang): Yes, including the captain.

**（依次对可疑旅客座位区域及卫生间、客舱整体、货舱消毒）**

(The seating area where the suspected infected passengers were seated, the lavatory, the entire cabin and the cargo hold are disinfected in turn)

**检疫关员（小王）：** 客舱终末消毒已完成。请关闭机舱门。

Officer (Xiao Wang): The terminal disinfection of the cabin has been completed. Please close the cabin doors.

**机长：**门关好了。我们需要等候多久？

Captain: The doors are closed. How long should we wait?

**检疫关员（小王）：**现在是下午 3：20。按照消毒方案，消毒液完全发挥作用需要 30 分钟，也就是说下午 3：50 以后才可以开启舱门。

Officer (Xiao Wang): It's 3:20 pm. According to the disinfection scheme, it takes 30 minutes for the disinfectant to become fully effective, which means that you can't open the cabin doors until 3:50 pm.

**乘务长：**好的。

Chief Attendant: Okay.

**检疫关员（小王）：**货舱也要进行消毒。在消毒液完全发挥作用后才能装卸货物。

Officer (Xiao Wang): The cargo hold should be disinfected too. Do not load or unload goods until the disinfectant has fully worked.

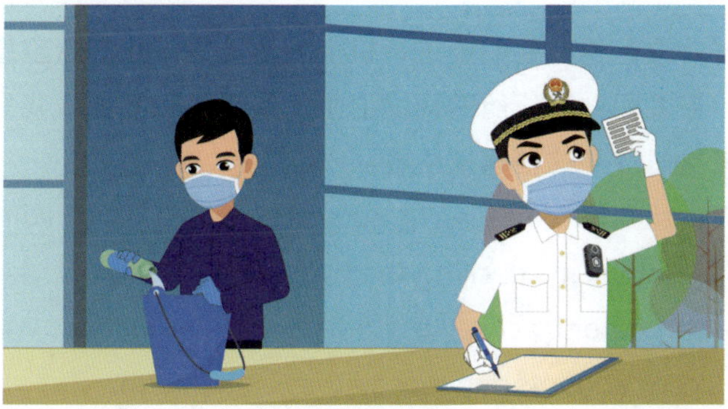

**机长：**也是 30 分钟吗？

Captain: It will take 30 minutes, right?

**检疫关员（小王）：**是的，您说得对。

Officer (Xiao Wang): Yes, you're right.

**(30 分钟后）**

(30 minutes later)

**检疫关员（小王）：** 终末消毒已完成。我们会为您出具证书。现在可以开始卸货了。

Officer (Xiao Wang): The terminal disinfection has been completed. We'll issue a certificate to you. Unloading of goods can start now.

**乘务长：** 好的。非常感谢您！

Chief Attendant: Great. Thank you very much!

**检疫关员（小王）：** 不客气！

Officer (Xiao Wang): You're welcome!

## 第三节 日常卫生监督
## SECTION III ROUTINE SUPERVISION OF HYGIENE

**检疫关员：** 您好，乘务长，我们要进行机上卫生监督。我们希望您能配合我们一起检查配餐间、卫生间、客货舱的环境卫生，饮用水和配餐。我们还会检查机上有没有蟑螂、老鼠、蚊子这些病媒生物。

Officer: Hello, Chief Attendant, we're going to check flight hygiene. We expect you to cooperate with us in checking the hygiene of the galley, the lavatories, the cockpit and the cargo hold, as well as potable water and food. We'll also check if there are cockroaches, rodents and mosquitoes on the flight.

**乘务长：** 没问题。我现在要做什么？

Chief Attendant: No problem. What can I do now?

**检疫关员：** 让我先看一下机组成员的健康证和卫生培训记录。

Officer: Let me take a look at the crew's health certificates and hygiene training records first.

**乘务长：** 好的，机组成员上岗前都体检过。这是他们的健康证。他们需要等到卫生培训合格后才能上岗。这是记录。

Chief Attendant: Okay, the crew have all had physical examinations. Here are their health certificates. They're not allowed to take up their jobs until they've completed hygiene training. Here are the records.

**检疫关员：** 您看这位乘务员的健康证快到期了。请提醒他及时去换证。

Officer: This flight attendant's health certificate is about to expire. Please remind him to have it renewed.

**乘务长：** 好的，我马上提醒他。

Chief Attendant: Sure, I'll do it.

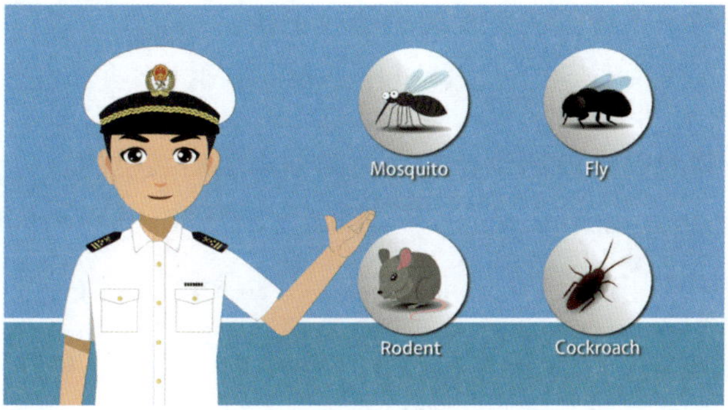


**检疫关员：** 证件和培训记录都没问题。我们先去检查配餐间。

Officer: The certificates and training records are in good order. Let us check the galley first.

**乘务长：** 好的。您随我来。这里是我们的配餐间。

Chief Attendant: Sure. Please follow me. This is our galley.

**检疫关员：** 今天机上准备了哪些餐食？

Officer: What food has been prepared today?

**乘务长：** 主食有鲜虾三文鱼芦笋沙拉、白酱鸡肉通心粉、咕咾肉盖饭。餐后水果是苹果、蓝莓，还有一些小饼干和蛋糕。

Chief Attendant: The main courses are fresh shrimp, salmon and asparagus salads, chicken macaroni mixed with white sauce, and rice topped with sweet and sour pork. The dessert fruits are apples and blueberries, there're also some small biscuits and cakes.

**检疫关员：**配回程餐了吗？

Officer: Have you prepared the meals for the return journey?

**乘务长：**没有。单程飞行就需要 5 个多小时，回程要等到明天，到时候本地的航食企业会供餐。

Chief Attendant: No. A one-way journey takes just a little over five hours, and the return journey is tomorrow, when a local airline caterer will supply the meals.

**检疫关员：**让我看一下今天的餐食装机验收记录。

Officer: Let me take a look at the acceptance record of today's meal loading.

**乘务长：**给您。餐食是在航班预计起飞时间前半小时装机的。

Chief Attendant: Here you are. Meals are loaded onto the plane half an hour before the scheduled departure time.

**检疫关员：**让我看看……今天飞机延误了半小时，直到上午 9:20 餐食才装机。到现在差不多 7 小时。餐食是放在哪里保存？

Officer: Let me have a look... Today the flight was delayed for half an hour, and the meals weren't loaded onboard until 9:20 am. It's been almost seven hours. Where do you keep the meals?

**乘务长：**在这个冷藏箱内。

Chief Attendant: Inside this refrigerated storage box.

**（一名关员正在使用测温仪检查餐食表面温度）**

(An Officer is checking the surface temperature of the meals with a thermometer)

**检疫关员：**乘务长，您看，这个餐食箱虽然温度设定在 10℃，但是实际餐食表面温度已经达到 13℃了。机上餐食的保存温度要低于 10℃，而且不超过 12 小时。如果使用干冰冷藏存放，时间不能超过 4 小时，否则食物，特别是三文鱼、虾这些冷食海鲜将会变质。

Officer: Chief Attendant, take a look, the temperature of this meal storage box is set at 10℃, but the real surface temperature of the meals is as high as 13℃. In-flight meals should be kept at a temperature below 10℃ and for no more than 12 hours. When dry ice is used for refrigeration, the meals should be kept for no more than four hours; otherwise, the food, especially the cold seafood like salmons and shrimps, will turn sour.

**乘务长：**是我们疏忽了。可能是这台机器年久保养不当。我马上报告公司检修。

Chief Attendant: We were so careless. Maybe the machine hasn't been properly serviced for a long time. I'll ask my company to check the machine right away.

**（查看烤箱）**

(Looking into the oven)

**检疫关员：**烤箱里还有食物没拿出来吗？

Officer: Is some food left inside the oven?

**乘务长：**啊，我很抱歉。餐食加热完之后，有几个机组成员没有吃，留在了烤箱里……我这就将这些剩余的餐食装袋妥善处理掉。

Chief Attendant: Ah, I'm very sorry. Some crews didn't eat the meals after they were heated, leaving them in the oven... I'll bag up these leftovers for proper disposal.

**检疫关员：**您一般是怎么处理加热后剩余的餐食和未开封的餐食？

Officer: What do you usually do with heated leftovers and unopened meals?

**乘务长：**公司要求未开封的餐食和已开封的剩余餐食，每航次后都必须作为废弃物处理。我们也会提醒旅客餐食不能带下飞机。这些都一起装袋后封扎好放到带盖垃圾桶里，航后处理。

Chief Attendant: We're required to dispose of unopened meals and leftovers as waste after flight. We also ask the passengers not to take the meals off the plane. We bag up and put them in a covered waste bin for disposal after the flight.

**检疫关员：** 做得很好。这个储水箱的水会提供给旅客饮用吗？

Officer: Pretty good. Do you offer water from this tank to passengers?

**乘务长：** 一般都给旅客提供瓶装水，但是如果旅客要求喝热水、茶或者咖啡，我们会把储水箱里的水加热后提供给他们饮用。

Chief Attendant: We usually offer bottled water to passengers, but if a passenger ask for hot water, tea or coffee, we'll heat water from the tank and give it to him.

**检疫关员：** 储水箱的水多久会换一次？

Officer: How often do you change the water in the tank?

**乘务长：** 每个航次飞完都会将储水箱里的水全部排空，起飞前再向水箱里加入清洁水。

Chief Attendant: We drain the water in the tank after flight and add freshwater to the tank before take off.

**检疫关员：** 储水箱平时是怎么清洗和消毒的？让我看一下工作记录。

Officer: How do you clean and disinfect the tank? Let me take a look at the work records.

**乘务长：** 给您。公司要求储水箱每周清洗和消毒一次，出水口处的过滤器每两周更换一次。

Chief Attendant: Here you are. We're required to clean and disinfect the tank once a week, and replace the filter at the outlet every two weeks.

**检疫关员：** 消毒记录都很清楚。机上会给旅客提供冰块吗？

Officer: The disinfection records are in good order. Do you offer ice cubes to passengers?

**乘务长：** 有的，都是由配餐公司统一配送上机，放在这个冰盒里。

Chief Attendant: Yes, they're loaded onto the plane by the caterer and kept in this ice box.

**检疫关员：** 要注意冰块不要跟其他的食物混放在一起，取冰用的冰铲也不能这样随意放在台面上，这样容易被细菌污染，并造成旅客腹泻。

Officer: Be careful not to mix ice cubes with other food items, and do not place the ice shovel on the table like this, because it will be contaminated by bacteria and cause diarrhea among passengers.

**乘务长：**好的。我们将再次对乘务员进行标准操作程序的培训。

Chief Attendant: All right. We'll train our flight attendants again in the standard operating procedures.

**检疫关员：**总的来说，配餐间卫生状况不错。食物、餐具都能分类存放。地板、台面没有明显的污渍、杂物、鼠迹或者蟑螂。包装零食生产日期也都在有效期内。但是，工作人员应该更严格地遵守标准操作程序。

Officer: On the whole, hygiene in the galley is pretty good. Food and tableware are stored by category. The floors and tables are free of stains, odds and ends, rodent or cockroach droppings. The packaged snacks are also well within their expiration dates. However, the staff should follow the standard operating procedures more strictly.

**乘务长：**好的。谢谢您指出这个问题。

Chief Attendant: All right. Thank you for pointing out the problem.

**检疫关员：**我们想采集一些水样进行检测，包括刚刚说的饮用水和冰块。（采样完成）好了，乘务长，一起去看看卫生间的情况吧。

Officer: We want to take some water samples for testing, including the potable water and ice cubes we just talked about. (Sampling completed) We're done here, Chief Attendant, let's check the lavatory.

**（地点：卫生间）**

(Location: Lavatory)

**检疫关员：**卫生间卫生做得不错。干净、整洁，没有异味。手边备有洗消剂，洗手池、镜子、垃圾桶和地面都很干净，没有积水。

Officer: The lavatory looks nice. It's clean, tidy and odor-free. Decontaminants are kept on hand. The washbasin, mirror, trash can and floor are all clean and free of standing water.

**乘务长：** 是的，公司的员工手册里对各个区域的卫生都有严格要求。我们还定期往污水箱投放消毒剂，航后统一进行废弃物处理。

Chief Attendant: Yes, our employee handbook has strict requirements for the hygiene of each area. We also put disinfectants into the sewage tank regularly, and carry out sewage treatment after flight.

**检疫关员：** 做得不错。再去客舱看看吧。

Officer: You've done a good job. Let's check out the cabin.

**乘务长：** 好的。

Chief Attendant: Okay.

**（地点：客舱）**

(Location: Cabin)

**检疫关员：** 乘务长，这些座椅头垫多久更换一次？您看这里有块明显的污渍。

Officer: Chief Attendant, how often do you change the headrests? You can see there is a distinct stain here.

**乘务长：** 不好意思，是我们清洁不到位。我们一般一个星期左右会更换一次。

Chief Attendant: Sorry, they haven't been properly cleaned. We usually change the headrests once a week or so.

**检疫关员：** 像座椅头垫、拖鞋、耳机、毛毯这些公用物品要定期消毒。尽量保证一航次一更换。

Officer: Communal items like headrests, slippers, earphones and blankets should be disinfected regularly. Try to use new ones for each flight.

**乘务长：** 好的。

Chief Attendant: All right.

**(海关关员进行微小气候和空气质量检测)**

(Customs Officers performing microclimate and air quality tests)

**乘务长:** 请问这些仪器是做什么用的?

Chief Attendant: What's this instrument for?

**检疫关员:** 这个是微小气候检测仪。简单来说就是通过测量机上的温度、湿度、CO、$CO_2$、照度、噪声和飞机上的风速，帮助我们了解机舱内的环境卫生情况是否符合要求。

Officer: This is a microclimate tester. We use it to measure the temperature, humidity, CO, $CO_2$, illuminance, noise and air speed on the aircraft, so that we can find out whether environmental hygiene in the cabin is up to standard.

**乘务长:** 明白了。

Chief Attendant: I see.

**检疫关员:** 乘务长，您看这边有几只蚊子在飞。起飞前喷过杀虫剂吗?

Officer: Chief Attendant, look, a few mosquitoes are flying around. Did you spray insecticide before take off?

**乘务长:** 哎呀，真的！我们有喷杀虫剂。是不是喷太少了有几只漏网之鱼?

Chief Attendant: Oh, my goodness! We did spray insecticide. Is it that we sprayed too little to kill them all?

**检疫关员:** 有这个可能。您平时用的什么杀虫剂？每次一般用多少？罐子拿给我看看。

Officer: Maybe. What insecticide do you usually use? And how much do you usually use each time? Please let me take a look at the cans.

**乘务长:** 给您。这两个空罐子是这个航班喷完的。

Chief Attendant: Here you are. We used up these two cans on this flight.

**检疫关员:** 我看看。嗯，杀虫剂成分是符合要求的。这是一架窄体机，用这个剂量看起来也没问题。是什么时候喷的呢？旅客登机前还是登机后?

Officer: Let me take a look. Well, the ingredients are fine. This is a narrow-body aircraft, so the volume of spray is okay. When did you spray the insecticide? Before or after boarding?

**乘务长：**我们在旅客登机前喷的，否则，旅客会投诉。

Chief Attendant: We sprayed before boarding; otherwise, passengers would complain.

**检疫关员：**给我看看您是怎么使用的。

Officer: Show me how you used it.

**乘务长：**这样。（演示喷除虫剂）

Chief Attendant: Like this. (Making a demonstration)

**检疫关员：**您看，问题就出在这儿。喷洒前，您要打开顶部和侧壁的行李柜，喷的时候要尽量从高处喷雾，以保证气雾均匀覆盖。还有，您喷洒的速度太快了。放慢速度大约每秒一排。

Officer: Well, that's the problem. Before spraying, you should open the overhead and side compartments, and you should start to spray high up, so that the droplets can cover the surface evenly. Also, you sprayed too fast. Go slower, passing one row per second or so.

**乘务长：**明白了。

Chief Attendant: I see.

**检疫关员：**（指着沟槽）喷洒时要特别注意这些缝隙、沟槽，它们通常是昆虫的藏身之处。除了客舱、货舱，也要确保喷雾覆盖到卫生间、配餐间、衣柜、储物柜、机组休息区。

Officer: (Pointing to the crevices) When you're spraying, pay close attention to the voids and crevices as they are common hideouts for insects. Besides the cabin and cargo hold, make sure the spray covers the lavatory, galley, wardrobes, lockers, and crew rest area.

**乘务长：**好的，我们会注意的。

Chief Attendant: Okay, we'll see to that.

**检疫关员：**除虫的时候，空调和风扇是关掉还是开着的？

Officer: Did you turn off the air-conditioners and fans or keep them running during insect removal?

**乘务长：**都是开着的。

Chief Attendant: We kept them running.

**检疫关员：**除虫期间飞机的空调系统必须关闭，喷洒后再关闭 5 分钟，否则除虫的效果会大打折扣。

Officer: The air-conditioning system must be shut down during insect removal and for five more minutes after spraying; otherwise, the effect of the insecticide would be seriously reduced.

**乘务长：**明白了。

Chief Attendant: I see.

**检疫关员：**乘务长，机上发现了数量较多的蚊子，它们是可能传播疾病的病媒生物，飞机必须进行除虫。我们会给您出具检验检疫处理通知书。

Officer: Chief Attendant, quite a few mosquitoes have been spotted and they're likely to cause the transmission of disease, insect removal must be carried out on the plane. We'll issue a Notification of Inspection and Quarantine Treatment to you.

**乘务长：**好的。我马上通知检疫处理公司。

Chief Attendant: All right. I'll contact the quarantine treatment company right away.

**检疫关员：**除虫完成前不能卸货。

Officer: Do not unload any cargo before insect removal is completed.

**乘务长：**好的，我会注意。

Chief Attendant: Okay, I'll see to that.

**（除虫已完成）**

(Insect removal completed)

**检疫关员：** 我们会为您签发证书。现在您可以安排卸货了。

Officer: We'll issue the certificate to you. Now you arrange for cargo unloading.

**乘务长：** 好的。非常感谢！

Chief Attendant: Great. Thank you very much!

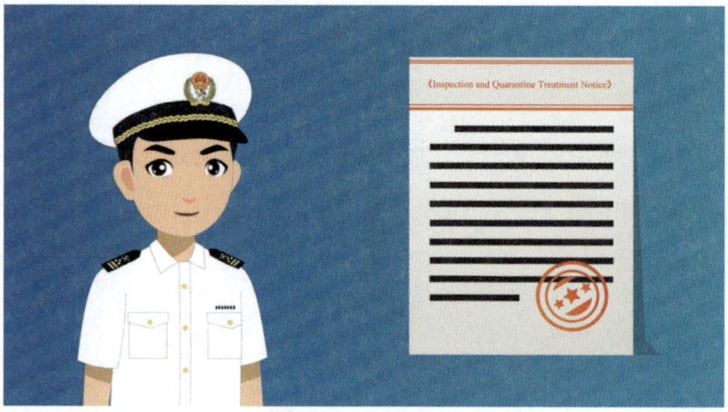

# 第二部分　船舶登临检疫

PART II　BOARDING AND QUARANTINE OF SHIPS

## 第一节 单证检查和健康信息询问

SECTION I DOCUMENTATION REVIEW AND OBTAINING MARITIME HEALTH INFORMATION

**检疫关员：** 船长，您好，我们是 XX 海关关员，根据《中华人民共和国国境卫生检疫法》，我们需要对您管理的这艘船进行登轮检查，请您或船医配合我们的工作。

Officer: Hello, Captain, we're Officers of XX Customs. Under the *Frontier Health and Quarantine Law of the People's Republic of China*, we need to inspect your ship, and we expect you or the ship doctor to cooperate with us.

**船长：** 很高兴见到您。非常欢迎您来检查。

Captain: Glad to see you. Welcome onboard for the inspection.

**检疫关员：** 船长，刚才登船时我们看到您的船舶悬挂着黄旗，但现在已经是夜间了，根据中国法律，您应该开启垂直的三盏红灯。

Officer: Captain, upon boarding the ship just now, we saw your ship flying a yellow flag, but because it is night now, under Chinese law, you should turn on three vertical red lights.

**船长：** 好的。船舶入境是傍晚，我们就还是挂了黄旗。下次我们一定注意。我现在马上安排人员去将三盏红色信号灯打开。

Captain: Okay. We arrived at dusk, so we hoisted a yellow flag. We'll be careful next time. I'll send someone to turn on the three red signal lights right now.

**检疫关员：** 没关系，船长，请出示航海健康申报书、最新的船舶免予卫生控制措施证书、船员名单、港序列表、旅客名单、疫苗接种名单等单证。

Officer: Okay, Captain, please show us your Maritime Declaration of Health, latest Ship Sanitation Control Exemption Certificate, Crew List, Ports of Call List, Passenger List and Vaccination List , etc.

**船长：** 我们已经准备好这些文件，请查阅。

Captain: We have these documents ready for your inspection.

**检疫关员：** 船舶航行途中是否有出现发热、咳嗽、呼吸困难、腹泻、呕吐等传染病症状的船员或旅客？是否有船员下地就医？是否能出示你们的医疗记录本以便我们核实？

Officer: Did any crew or passenger have symptoms of infection, such as fever, cough, difficulty in breathing, diarrhea or vomiting, during the voyage? Did any crew leave the ship for medical treatment? Would you please show us your Medical Logbook so that we can verify the information?

**船长：** 这是我们的医疗记录本。您可以看到，航行途中我们每天两次量体温，每个船员都很健康。船公司也要求我们船员有健康问题要及时上报。

Captain: Here is our Medical Logbook. As you can see, we took temperature of every crew twice a day during the voyage. All the crew are in good health condition. The shipowner also requires us to report any health problems immediately.

**检疫关员：** 根据你们的港序列表，你们的船舶在 2 周前挂靠过 F 港。F 港作为近期呼吸道传染病疫情的流行区，你们的船员是否有下地，是否有接触过当地的人员？

Officer: According to your Ports of Call List, your ship called at Port F two weeks ago. Port F has been an endemic area of respiratory infectious diseases recently. Did any of your crew come ashore and have contact with local people?

**船长：** 没有。我们的船公司不允许我们在 F 港下地，而且要求在 F 港作业期间必须奉行“非必要不接触”的政策。

Captain: No. The shipowner did not allow us to come ashore at Port F and required us to follow the policy of “nocontact unless absolutely necessary” when we called at Port F.

**检疫关员：** 船上是否发现病媒生物，如蝇类、蟑螂、鼠、蚊子？是否出现鼠类异常死亡情况？

Officer: Did you find any rodents or insects, such as flies, cockroaches, and mosquitoes onboard? And did you notice any unusual deaths of rodents?

**船长：** 没有发现这类情况。我们在港期间每两天消毒一次，航行途中每周消毒一次。我要保证船员的身体健康。

Captain: No, we didn't. We performed disinfection every two days when we docked at a port and once a week during the voyage. I make sure the crew are in good health.

**检疫关员：** 船长，我们需要查看压载水申报单、压载水管理计划、压载水记录本。

Officer: Captain, we need to check your Ballast Water Report, Ballast Water Management Plan and Ballast Water Logbook.

**船长：** 在这里。

Captain: Here you are.

**检疫关员：** 你们是在这里排放压载水吗？

Officer: Will you discharge ballast water here?

**船长：** 不，我们不会。我们通常在公海排放压载水。我们很少在港口这么做。

Captain: No, we will not. We usually discharge the ballast water on the open sea. We rarely do it at a port.

**检疫关员：** 我们需要查看您的垃圾管理计划和垃圾记录本。

Officer: We need to check your Garbage Management Plan and Garbage Logbook.

**船长：** 在这里。

Captain: Here you are.

**检疫关员：** 你们准备卸载垃圾吗？

Officer: Are you going to discharge the garbage?

**船长：** 我们计划在这里卸载垃圾。等你们检疫完毕，经过卫生处理后，就把垃圾卸下去。

Captain: We plan to discharge the garbage here. We'll do it after you've completed the inspection and after the garbage has undergone sanitary treatment.

**检疫关员：** 食物是从哪个港口装载的？请给我们一份食品清单。

Officer: At which port did you load the food? Please give us a copy of your Food Supply List.

**船长：** 我们在新加坡带的食物基本吃光了，在这里还需要重新补给。这是食品清单和入库台账。

Captain: The food supply we took in Singapore has almost run out and so we need to resupply here. This is our Food Supply List and Food Storage Ledger.

**检疫关员：** 食物确实快用光了。文件审核到此为止。请您召集所有船员进行测温。

Officer: The food supply really runs out fast. We're done reviewing the documents. Please call your crew up for temperature measurement.

**船长：** 好的。（广播）所有船员请到船长办公室集合。

Captain: Okay. (Intercom announcement) All crew please come to the Captain's Office.

**检疫关员：** 所有船员按船员名单顺序一个接一个进来测温。船长请协助我们登记，谢谢。

Officer: The crew are expected to come in one by one in the order of their names on the Crew List. Captain, please help us with the registration , thank you.

**船长：** 好的。我是第一个。

Captain: Sure. I'll be the first one.

**检疫关员：** 您好！红外温度计提示您的体温超过了 37℃。我们需要对您进行体温复测。请把水银温度计夹在您的腋下，5 分钟后取下。

Officer: Hello! The infrared thermometer shows your temperature is over 37℃. We need to take your temperature again. Please keep the mercury thermometer under your armpit for five minutes.

**船员 A：** 我刚刚从机舱上来，满头大汗。能不能先休息一下？

Crew A: I've just got out of the engine room, and I'm sweating buckets. Can I take a rest for a while?

**检疫关员：** 好的。您先休息一下，再测体温。

Officer: Okay. Take a short rest before having your temperature taken.

**检疫关员：** 36.8℃，体温正常，您可以返回继续工作。机舱温度高，要注意休息。

Officer: It's 36.8℃, your body temperature is fine, you can go back to work. It's hot in the engine room, make sure you get enough rest.

**船员 A：** 好的。谢谢！

Crew A: All right. Thank you!

## 第二节 现场检查
## SECTION II ON-SITE INSPECTION

### 场景一 厨房
### SCENE 1: GALLEY

**检疫关员：** 您好，大厨，我们要检查厨房。请出示清洁时间表和记录，以及杀虫剂使用记录。

Officer: Hello, Chief Cook, we need to inspect the galley. Please show us the cleaning schedule and log, as well as the insecticide application log.

**大厨：** 清洁记录、杀虫剂使用记录都在这里。当发现有害虫的时候，我会在第一时间杀灭它们。

Chief Cook: Here are the cleaning and insecticide application logs. I wipe out the insects whenever I find them.

**检疫关员：** 这个垃圾桶的盖子没盖好，有几只苍蝇从桶里面飞出来。虽然你们有杀虫剂，也有做记录，但是从现场可以看出你们的实际操作能力还需进一步提高。你们可以通过代理联系专业公司进行除虫处理。

Officer: This waste bin is not properly covered, and a few flies have just flied out of it. You do have insecticides and keep logs, but judging from what we see here, there is still much room for improvement. You may contact a PCO company through an agent for insect removal.

**大厨：** 我记住了。

Chief Cook: I'll do that.

**检疫关员：** 您在进行不同的任务之间会洗手吗？当您制作生食和熟食时，会分开使用砧板吗？

Officer: Do you wash your hands between tasks? Do you use separate chopping boards for raw and cooked food?

**大厨：** 当然，我会。生熟分开很重要。这是生食的刀和砧板，这边是熟食的。

Chief Cook: Yes, I do. It's very important to separate raw and cooked food items. These are the cutters and the chopping boards for raw food, and those are for cooked food.

**检疫关员：** 最近一段时间您有生过病吗？

Officer: Have you been ill recently?

**大厨：** 没有。

Chief Cook: No , I haven't.

**检疫关员：** 让我们到供餐间看看。这个桌子上没有防护罩，被放在那个凳子上了。请把它盖到食物上面。

Officer: Let's go to the galley. This table doesn't have a protective cover. The cover is placed on that stool instead. Please put it over the food.

**大厨：** 这是我的失误。

Chief Cook: It's my fault.

**检疫关员：** 厨房有食品温度计吗？

Officer: Do you have a food thermometer?

**大厨：** 有的，在这里。

Chief Cook: Yes, it's here.

**检疫关员：** 检查完毕。感谢您的配合！

Officer: We're done with the inspection. Thank you for cooperation!

**大厨：** 不用谢！

Chief Cook: You're welcome.

## 场景二 食品仓库

SCENE 2: FOOD STORAGE

**检疫关员：** 大厨，我们已经检查完厨房的卫生。我们想看看存储室的卫生状况是否符合要求，能给我带路吗？

Officer: Chief Cook, we've completed our inspection of the galley. We'd like to see if hygiene in the storage rooms is up to standard, would you please take me to the galley?

**大厨：** 好的。请跟我走。

Chief Cook: Sure. Please follow me.

**检疫关员：**稍等，先看一下储藏室的温度控制系统。

Officer: Hold on a second. Let's take a look at the temperature control system for the storage rooms.

**大厨：**这个屏幕显示的是我们各个库房的温度。肉和鱼保存温度低于 −18℃。这是温度记录本。

Chief Cook: This screen displays the temperatures of our storage rooms. Meat and fish are kept at a temperature below −18℃. This is the temperature logbook.

**检疫关员：**这包大米长虫了，不能再吃了。你们应该把它扔掉，为每一名船员的健康负责。在扔弃之前，请允许我们采样。

Officer: This bag of rice is wormy and can no longer be eaten. You should have disposed of it as you're responsible for the crew's health. We would like to take a sample.

**大厨：**好的，请便。

Chief Cook: Sure, go ahead please.

**检疫关员：**大米应该放到架子上，而不是让它靠在墙上。

Officer: The rice should be kept on the shelf rather than be placed against the wall.

**大厨：**大米从架子上拿下来忘记放回去了。谢谢您的提醒。

Chief Cook: We forgot to put it back after taking it down. Thank you for reminding us.

**检疫关员：**您看，这箱咖啡有效期到 2022 年 5 月 31 日，已经过期了。请尽快把它们清理掉。

Officer: Look, the expiration date of this box of coffee is May 31, 2022, and it has expired. Please get rid of it quickly.

**大厨：**好的。服务员，过来把这箱咖啡搬出去。

Chief Cook: Okay. Waiter, come and move this box of coffee out.

**检疫关员：**食品仓库的卫生检查到此为止。感谢您的配合！

Officer: We're done with our inspection of food warehouse hygiene. Thank you for your cooperation!

**大厨：** 好的。您说的几个问题我会及时整改。
Chief Cook: All right. I'll take immediate action to fix the problems you've just pointed out.

## 场景三 医疗室

SCENE 3: HOSPITAL

**检疫关员：** 大副，您好！医疗室在哪？能带我去看看吗？
Officer: Hello, Chief Officer! Where is the hospital located? Would you please take me there?

**大副：** 您好！医疗室在 B 层，请跟我来。
Chief Officer: Hello! The hospital is located on B Deck. Please follow me.

**检疫关员：** 这条船的船医是谁？能把他的培训执照给我看一下吗？
Officer: Who is the ship doctor? Could you show me his training license?

**大副：** 船上三副以上的船员都有经过相关的海上医疗与急救培训。他们具备海上急救的基本常识，也能够熟练地使用远程医疗救助服务。这是我们的培训证书。
Chief Officer: Crew above the rank of third officer have all received maritime medical and first aid training. They possess the fundamental knowledge of maritime first aid, and are able to use telemedical assistance services skillfully. Here are our training certificates.

**检疫关员：** 好的，让我看看。你们的医疗室设计合理，医疗器材和设备很齐全，环境也很干净。你们的药品是从哪里购买的？有没有合格证明？
Officer: Okay, let's take a look. This hospital is well designed and has a full range of medical instruments and equipment. It is very clean here, too. Where did you purchase the medicines? And do they come with quality certificates?

**大副：** 请看，这是药品清单和药品合格证明。这个黑色箱子装的是过期药品，上面有标识。

Chief Officer: Here are the medicine list and the quality certificates. Expired medicines are placed in this black box, and the box is clearly marked.

**检疫关员：** 好的。请把你们的用药记录给我看看。

Officer: Good. Please show me your medical record.

**大副：** 没问题，这是用药记录。

Chief Officer: Sure, here it is.

**检疫关员：** 用药记录显示昨天有人用过药。能说明一下具体情况吗？

Officer: The record shows that someone was given some medicines yesterday. Would you please tell me what the situation was?

**大副：** 轮机长干活撞到腰了，有点肿，但不是很严重，他仍然像往常一样工作。

Chief Officer: The Chief Engineer hurt his waist while working—a little swollen, but not very serious, and he still works as usual.

**检疫关员：** 能把他叫过来吗？

Officer: Can you call him up?

**轮机长：** 您好，我那天在机舱连接污油管，下楼梯时不小心磕到腰了。

Chief Engineer: Hello! I was connecting the sludge pipe in the engine room, and I accidentally hit my waist while going down the stairs.

**检疫关员：** 让我看看。腰部又红又肿。您有发热或其他症状吗？

Officer: Let me have a look. It is reddish and swollen. Do you have a fever or other symptoms?

**轮机长：** 没有，我很健康，照常工作。

Chief Engineer: No. I'm fit and healthy, and I work as usual.

**检疫关员：** 好的，还是要小心，不要剧烈活动。大副，你们得定期清洁医疗室。

清洁记录在哪？

Officer: Good. Be careful anyway, and avoid strenuous activities. Chief Officer, you have to clean the hospital regularly. Where is the cleaning record?

**大副：** 这是清洁记录。我们会定期清洁医疗室。保持医疗室的卫生清洁非常重要。

Chief Officer: Here it is. We clean the hospital regularly. It's very important to keep the hospital clean.

**检疫关员：** 你们医疗室的垃圾桶是黑色的。按规定，医疗废弃物应该放在黄色垃圾桶里面并进行标示。

Officer: You've got a black waste bin here. According to regulations, medical waste should be placed in a yellow bin and properly marked.

**大副：** 我们会更换一个黄色垃圾桶，专门用来装医疗废弃物。

Chief Officer: We'll get a yellow waste bin and use it for medical waste only.

**检疫关员：** 好的。检查完毕。谢谢！

Officer: Okay. We're done with the inspection. Thank you!

**大副：** 不用谢！

Chief Officer: You're welcome!

## 场景四 饮用水

SCENE 4: POTABLE WATER

**检疫关员：** 船长，您好！能告诉我船上有几套供水系统吗？

Officer: Hello, Captain, would you tell me how many water supply systems you have onboard?

**船长：** 我们有 3 套供水系统：饮用水、机器用水及消防用水。它们之间是相互独立的。

Captain: We have three water supply systems: potable water, machine water, and firefighting water. They're independent of one another.

**检疫关员：**清洁水和饮用水之间是相连通的吗？它们有共用管道吗？

Officer: What about the connection between clean water and potable water? Do they share pipes?

**船长：**不，不共用。它们之间是独立的。

Captain: No , they don't. They're separated from each other.

**检疫关员：**我们检查的重点是饮用水。请给我们一份你们的水质分析报告、水安全计划和医学日志。

Officer: The most important item to inspect is potable water. Please give us a copy of your Water Analysis Report, Water Safety Plan and Medical Logbook.

**船长：**稍等。我把饮用水检测报告和饮用水安全计划找出来给你们。找到了，给您。

Captain: Just a minute. I'll get the Potable Water Test Report and Potable Water Safety Plan for you. Here you are.

**船长：**船上饮用水是二副管理，这是他的培训证书。我们一个月对饮用水检测一次并记录检测结果。这是我们的记录。

Captain: The Second Officer is in charge of potable water, this is his training certificate. We test potable water once a month and record the test results. Here is our record.

**检疫关员：**能给我们看看你们的检测设备吗？

Officer: Would you please show us your testing equipment?

**船长：**没问题。这是余氯检测设备，这是比色卡，这是最近一次检测的照片。

Captain: Sure. This is the residual chlorine testing equipment, this is the color chart, and this is the photo of the last test.

**检疫关员：**你们自制的饮用水是从哪里来的，是来自港口还是公海？

Officer: Where do you get water to make potable water, from the open sea or from a port?

**船长**：我们都是在公海取水，这样更安全。

Captain: We fetch water from the open sea, it is safer.

**检疫关员**：做得对。当你们自制饮用水时，有没有安装消毒（比如自动加氯器）、矿化设备？

Officer: You do it right. Do you have disinfection equipment (such as automatic chlorinators) and mineralization equipment for making potable water?

**船长**：当然有。它们是必不可少的设备。

Captain: Certainly. They're essential equipment.

**检疫关员**：能不能带我们去看看你们的设备？你们的饮用水池多长时间清洗一次？

Officer: Would you please show us your equipment? How often do you clean your potable water pool?

**船长**：没问题，大副会带您过去看我们的设备。饮用水仓一年清洗一次，如果出现问题，我们会立即进行清洗。

Captain: Sure, the Chief Officer will show you our equipment. The potable water compartment is cleaned once a year, and if there's a problem, we'll do cleaning immediately.

**检疫关员**：现在能让我们去看看你们的消毒设备，同时对水温进行检测吗？

Officer: Now can you show us your disinfection equipment, are we also going to check the water temperature at the same time?

**船长**：好的，跟着大副走就行了。如果您还有任何其他问题，不要犹豫可以直接问大副。

Captain: Okay, just follow the Chief Officer. If you have any other questions, don't hesitate to ask the Chief Officer.

**检疫关员：** 好的，非常感谢！

Officer: Okay, thank you very much!

## 第三节 检疫结果判定及签证

## SECTION III INSPECTION RESULTS DETERMINATION AND CERTIFICATION GRANTING

**检疫关员：** 船长，您好，我们经过详细地检查，已经完成检疫流程。船舶在您的管理之下非常有序。我们在检查过程中发现的一些小问题已经向相关的人员提出来了，希望你们尽快整改。结合单证验核、现场检查等多方面结论，该船舶判定为非染疫船舶，不需要采取额外的检疫措施了。

Officer: Hello, Captain. We've completed the quarantine procedures with careful inspections. Your ship has been operating in an extremely orderly manner. We've found some minor problems during the inspections, and we've alerted your staff. We hope you'll fix them as soon as possible. Based on the conclusions from our document verification and onboard inspections, this ship is accredited as "non-infected", and no additional quarantine measures are necessary.

**船长：** 真是太好了！

Captain: That's wonderful!

**检疫关员：** 这是今天的检查记录单。如果您没有异议的话，请在这里签字并盖章。

Officer: This is today's inspection sheet. If you accept it, please sign and stamp on this column.

**船长：** 没问题！

Captain: Sure!

**检疫关员：** 这是船舶入境卫生检疫证书。请关闭检疫信号灯，船舶可以上下人员，装卸货物了。

Officer: Here is the Free Pratique. Please turn off the quarantine signal lights, and people are now allowed to get on or off the ship and load or unload goods.

**船长：**太棒了，谢谢你们。

Captain: Great, thank you very much.

**检疫关员：**不客气，再见。

Officer: You're welcome，goodbye.

**船长：**再见！

Captain: Goodbye!

# 第三章

CHAPTER III

# 突发公共卫生事件应急处置

RESPONDING TO A PUBLIC HEALTH EMERGENCY

# 第一部分　船舶（货轮）

PART I　SHIPS (CARGO SHIPS)

## 第一节 航海健康信息询问

SECTION I OBTAINING MARITIME HEALTH INFORMATION

**检疫关员：** 船长，您好，我们是中国海关关员。由于您的船舶申报有两名船员发热，所以要对你们的船舶实施登临检疫做进一步的检疫排查。希望您配合。

Officer: Hello, Captain, we're officers of China Customs. Since you declare that two members of your crew have a fever, we need to conduct quarantine inspections onboard. We hope you'll cooperate with us.

**船长：** 好的，我会全力配合。

Captain: Sure, I'll fully cooperate with you.

**检疫关员：** 请出示本航次的航海健康申报单。

Officer: Please show us the Maritime Declaration of Health for this voyage.

**船长：** 好的，给您。

Captain: Okay, here you are.

**检疫关员：** 根据航海健康申报单，在过去的 5 天里，5 名船员出现了畏寒、发热、头痛、肌肉酸痛等症状。请您具体描述一下情况。

Officer: According to the Maritime Declaration of Health, five crew members have developed symptoms, like chill, fever, headache and muscleache, over the past five days. Please give us a detailed account of the situation.

**船长：** 我请船上负责医疗的二副来向您介绍具体的情况。

Captain: I'll ask the Second Officer in charge of medical care onboard to give you more information.

**二副：** 大概 5 天前，船上的大厨告诉我，他出现了畏寒、发热、头痛的症状，我测了一下他的体温是 38.1℃。我就给他吃了退热药，现在他感觉好多了。

Second Officer: About five days ago, the ship's Chief Cook told me that he had symptoms like chills, fever and headache. I took his temperature, and it was 38.1℃. I gave him some antipyretics, and he feels better now.

**检疫关员：** 您把用药记录在医疗日志上了吗？能给我们看看医疗日志吗？

Officer: Did you record the medication in the Medical Logbook? Could you please show us the Medical Logbook?

**二副：** 服用的是扑热息痛。这是医疗日志，记录了我给他用药的时间。您可以看一下。

Second Officer: It was paracetamol. Here's the Medical Logbook, showing the time I handed him the medicines. You can have a look.

**检疫关员：** 医疗日志上记录了他在 12 小时后又出现了发热的症状，还服用了抗生素。

Officer: The Medical Logbook shows that he developed fever again 12 hours later and took antibiotics.

**二副：** 是的，吃退烧药只是暂时缓解，他的病情持续了好几天。

Second Officer: Yes, antipyretics provided only temporary relief, and his condition persisted for several days.

**检疫关员：** 其他船员呢？

Officer: What about other crew members?

**二副：** 其他 4 名有症状人员中，三副和水手长是在 3 天前出现的发热症状。昨天晚上，2 名高级水手（A、B）也出现了类似的症状。和大厨一样，他们也是服用了退热药和抗生素，效果也是一样。

Second Officer: Among the other four other symptomatic crew members, the Third Officer and the Bosun had a fever three days ago. Last night, two Able Seamen (A, B) also developed similar symptoms. Like the Chief Cook, they've also taken antipyretics and antibiotics, and the results are the same.

**检疫关员：**（对船长说）这些船员现在情况如何？

Officer: (Tell the Captain) How're these crew members now?

**船长：**他们被隔离在自己的宿舱内。今天早些时候，他们都测量了体温，结果显示还有发热症状。这是这几天的体温监测表。

Captain: They're isolated in their own rooms. Earlier today, they all had their temperature taken, and it shows that all of them still have fever symptoms. Here's the temperature measurement sheet for the past few days.

**检疫关员：**其他船员的情况如何？

Officer: What about the rest of the crew?

**船长：**其他船员身体健康，没有出现类似的症状。

Captain: The rest of the crew are in good health and show no similar symptoms.

## 第二节 船舶挂港信息调查
## SECTION II OBTAINING PORT ROTATION INFORMATION

**检疫关员：**船长，我们需要进一步了解船舶的航行情况。请给我们看一下船舶的航海日志和港序列表。

Officer: Captain, we need to know more about the voyage of the ship. Please show us the Nautical Logbook and the Ports of Call List.

**船长：**请稍等，给您。

Captain: Wait a second, here you are.

**检疫关员：** 船长，根据航海日志和船舶 A I S 轨迹查询，我们发现您在填报入境信息时，存在着漏报港序的情况。S 港口作为近期呼吸道传染病和蚊媒传染病重要的流行港口，您未在航海健康申报单中申报近 4 周内停靠过这个港口，这将影响我们对你们船舶风险的判断。

Officer: Captain, based on the Nautical Logbook and the AIS tracking results, we've found that some ports information is missing from your entry declaration. Port S is located in a major area hit by the recent outbreak of a respiratory infectious disease and a mosquito-borne infectious disease, you haven't declared that your ship has called at this port within the past four weeks in the Maritime Declaration of Health, and it will mislead our judgement of your vessel's risk.

**船长：** 对不起，这是我的疏忽。我忽视了申报单上信息的审核。我绝对无意隐瞒挂港信息。您知道的，现在的技术手段很方便，很容易就查到船舶的港序。我们的工作疏忽了，我为我们的疏忽道歉。

Captain: I apologize for my negligence. I neglected to check the information in the declaration. I have absolutely no intention to conceal any port rotation information. You know, given today's technology, it's very easy to find out the ship's ports of call. We were negligent in our work, I do apologize for our negligence.

**检疫关员：** 我们需要详细的船舶航线信息，还有近一个月以来船舶曾到达哪些港口。

Officer: We need detailed information about your ship's routing, as well as the ports your ship have called at over the past month.

**船长：** 我们沿地中海至欧洲航线航行。28 天前在欧洲的 H 港，15 天前通过了苏伊士运河，7 日前到了 S 港进行作业和补给。作业持续了 24 小时，3 月 15 日我们离开了 S 港。从那以后的一个月里，我们的船员都没有上岸，只有一些码头工人和船舶供应人员上了船。这是在舷梯口登记的相关记录。

Captain: We sailed on the Mediterranean-Europe route. We were at Port H in Europe 28 days ago, we passed through the Suez Canal 15 days ago, and we called at Port S for operations and supplies seven days ago. The operations lasted 24 hours, and we left Port S on March 15. For a month since then, none of our crew members has come ashore, and only some stevedores and ship supply guys have come onboard. Here's the visit or record.

**检疫关员：** 您是否记得看到过任何健康异常的人上船？

Officer: Do you remember seeing anyone coming onboard who appeared to have unusual health condition?

**船长：** 这是负责梯口值班的水手，由他向您介绍更多的信息。

Captain: This is the sailor on duty on the gangway, and he'll give you more information.

**值班水手：** 在欧洲港口时，除了引航员和工人外没有其他人员上船。在 S 港时，当天工人没有什么特别的印象，但有一名物料供应人员似乎有一些发热，但是我们没有检测他的体温。

Sailor on Duty: When we were at the European ports, no one boarded the ship except the pilots and workers. While at Port S, all workers looked quite normal, but a supply guy seemed to have a fever ; however, we didn't check his temperature.

**检疫关员：** 您怎么知道他发热了？

Officer: How did you know he had a fever?

**值班水手：** 因为他脸有点红，好像喝醉的样子，还在咳嗽。

Sailor on Duty: He looked flushed, as if he were drunk , and he was coughing.

**检疫关员：** 他是否进入了生活区？

Officer: Did he enter the accommodation area?

**值班水手：** 是的，进入了生活区，但应该只是从主层甲板走进办公室。

Sailor on Duty: Yes, he did, but he was likely to have walked into the office on the main deck only.

**检疫关员：** 他都和谁有过密切接触？

Officer: Whom did he have close contact with?

**值班水手：** 几乎全船都有接触，因为他向大家兜售了电话卡。

Sailor on Duty: Almost everyone onboard, because he was hawking phone cards.

**船长：** 这点我可以证实，因为我从他那儿购买了一张。

Captain: I can confirm this, because I bought one from him.

**检疫关员：** 他是否戴了口罩或手套等个人防护用品？

Officer: Did he wear personal protective equipment, such as a mask or gloves?

**值班水手：** 完全没有，没有任何的防护。

Sailor on Duty: None of these things.

**检疫关员：** 好的。还有其他补充吗？

Officer: Okay. Do you have anything to add?

**值班水手：** 没有了。

Sailor on Duty: Nope.

## 第三节 流行病学调查

## SECTION III CONDUCTING EPIDEMIOLOGICAL INVESTIGATION

**检疫关员：** 船长，根据我们所了解的，不能排除船上暴发传染病的可能性，需要做进一步的排查。请您做好配合。

Officer: Captain, to the best of our knowledge, we can't rule out the possibility of the outbreak of an infectious disease onboard, and further investigation is needed. Please cooperate with us.

**船长：** 我会全力配合好您的工作。

Captain: I'll fully cooperate with you.

**检疫关员：** 请给我一张船舶的楼层分布图，并标记患病船员的宿舱位置。

Officer: Please give me copy of the ship's floor general arrangement plan, with the location of the sick crew members' rooms marked on it.

**船长：** 这是我们的楼层分布图。大厨住在 B 层，两名高级水手在 C 层，他们的宿舱紧挨着。水手长住在 D 层，三副住在 E 层。

Captain: Here is our ship's floor general arrangement plan. The Chief Cook lives on Deck B, and the two Senior Sailors live on Deck C in rooms next to each other. The Bosun lives on Deck D, and the Third Officer lives on Deck E.

**检疫关员：** 他们在日常的工作过程中与他人密切接触的频率怎么样？

Officer: How often do they have close contact with others in their daily work?

**船长：** 因为都生活在船上，几乎大家每天都有密切接触，特别是水手。

Captain: Since they all live onboard, they have close contact with almost everyone else every day , especially the sailors.

**检疫关员：** 接触形式有哪些？ 面对面交谈吗？

Officer: In what ways? Face-to-face conversations?

**船长：** 近距离的交谈肯定是有的。更重要的是，在工作过程中身体接触是不可避免的。

Captain: Yes, there're such conversations. What's more, physical contact is unavoidable during work.

**检疫关员：** 我明白了，请确保这几名生病的船员继续在房间里等待，告诉他们不要紧张，保持平静。其他船员全部到医疗室等候。我们先测量其他船员的体温。请协助我们组织好船员按船员名单上的顺序一个接一个地过来测量体温。

Officer: I see. Please make sure these sick crew members stay in their rooms, and tell them not to be nervous but keep calm. Ask all the other crew members to wait in the hospital. We'll measure the other crew members' temperature first. Please help us get the crew members to come over one by one in the order of their names on the Crew List for temperature measurement.

**船长：** 好的。

Captain: Sure.

**（开始检测体温和医学巡查，检测结束后未发现异常）**

(Temperature measurement and medical inspection start, with no abnormality found upon completion)

## 第四节 有症状人员流行病学调查、医学检查和采样

## SECTION IV CONDUCTING EPIDEMIOLOGICAL INVESTIGATION, MEDICAL EXAMINATION AND SAMPLING FOR SYMPTOMATIC PERSONS

**检疫关员：** 船长，通过体温检测未发现其他船员有发热的症状。现在请带我们到那两名有症状船员的宿舱。

Officer: Captain, temperature measurement has shown no other crew members have fever symptoms. Please take us to the rooms of the two symptomatic crew members.

**船长：** 好的，我们先去哪一位的房间呢？

Captain: Okay, which one shall we go to first?

**检疫关员：** 先去大厨的房间，他是第一个出现症状的人。

Officer: The Chief Cook's room first, he was the first one to have symptoms.

**船长：** 好的。

Captain: All right.

**检疫关员：** 您好，大厨，我们是中国海关关员。我们需要对您的病情做进一步的了解。请您配合。

Officer: Hello, Chief Cook, we're officers of China Customs. We need to know more about your condition. Please cooperate with us.

**大厨：**好的。

Chief Cook: Sure.

**检疫关员：**请出示您的护照，并告诉我们您的姓名、出生日期、国籍、船上的职务。

Officer: Please show us your passport, and tell us your name, date of birth, nationality and job title on the ship.

**检疫关员：**现在人感觉如何？除了发热外还有没有什么特别的症状？

Officer: How do you feel now? Do you have any special symptoms other than fever?

**大厨：**现在仍然感觉有些发热。喉咙痛，偶尔会咳嗽。

Chief Cook: I still feel a little feverish. I have a sore throat and cough occasionally.

**检疫关员：**这是水银体温计。请在腋下夹紧，5 分钟后取出。我们有几个问题要问您，请您尽可能如实回答。您是什么时候开始感觉不舒服的？

Officer: Here's a mercury thermometer. Please keep it under your armpit for five minutes. We have a few questions for you, please answer them as truthfully as possible. When did you start feeling any discomfort?

**大厨：**大概 5 天前的半夜，1 点左右，我突然感到冷和头痛。后来，我就发热了，还有头痛和肌肉痛。

Chief Cook: About five days ago in the middle of the night, at about 1 o'clock, I suddenly had chills and a headache. Later, I had a fever, a headache and muscle pain.

**检疫关员：**当时发热到几度？

Officer: What was your temperature then?

**大厨：**我去找二副拿药。他量了我的体温，是 38.1℃。

Chief Cook: I asked the Second Officer for medication. He took my temperature, and it was 38.1℃.

**检疫关员：**您后来吃药了吗？

Officer: Did you take medicines later?

**大厨：**二副给了我退热药。我吃下去后，退热了，但 2 小时后又发热了。后面几天头不痛了，肌肉痛也有好转，但发热一直持续，也有一些喉咙痛。两天前我开始偶尔咳嗽。

Chief Cook: The Second Officer gave me antipyretics. I took the medicine, and my fever was gone, but it came back two hours later. In the next few days, my headache was gone and the muscle pain eased off, but my fever persists and I have a sore throat. I started coughing occasionally two days ago.

**检疫关员：**您觉得是什么原因导致了发病？

Officer: Do you have any idea what made you sick?

**大厨：**我觉得应该是我发病前一天下午在冻库里整理食物受凉了。我以前感冒很快就好了，但是这次特别久。

Chief Cook: I think I caught a cold on the afternoon of the day before I got sick when I was sorting out food in the cold storage room. I used to get over a cold rather quickly , but this time it's lasting longer.

**检疫关员：**在发病前几天里，有没有密切接触过什么外来的人员？

Officer: In the few days before you got sick, did you have close contact with any persons other than the crew?

**大厨：**在 S 港，我们有补给伙食，并与两名伙食供应人员有过密切接触。我们还检查了他们供应的食物。

Chief Cook: At Port S, we received food supplies and had close contact with two supply guys. We also checked the food they brought onboard.

**检疫关员：**您有没有注意这两名人员有没有不寻常的地方？

Officer: Did you notice anything unusual about them?

**大厨：**经您这么提醒，我想起他们其中有个人看起来很累，有一些发热，甚至在卸货的时候咳嗽了。我当时也没在意，还以为他是喝多了。

Chief Cook: Now that you mention it, I remember one of the guys looked very tired and a little feverish, and he even coughed while unloading the supplies. I didn't take it seriously , as I simply thought he was drunk.

**检疫关员：**您和他是否有过面对面交谈？您戴口罩了吗？

Officer: Did you have a face-to-face conversation with him? Were you wearing a mask?

**大厨：**在清点食物的时候有近距离的接触和交谈。我只戴了手套，没有戴口罩。

Chief Cook: I did have close contact and a conversation with him while checking the food supplies. I only wore gloves but no mask.

**检疫关员：**接触了多长时间？

Officer: How long did the contact last?

**大厨：**这次供应的食物比较多，我们花了 1 个多小时才接收完。

Chief Cook: We ordered plenty of food. It took us more than an hour to take delivery.

**检疫关员：**是否有供应活的或死的野生动物？

Officer: Did the food supplies include any wild animals, live or dead?

**大厨：**不可能会有。它们都是正常的鸡肉和牛肉。

Chief Cook: Absolutely not. They were just ordinary chicken and beef.

**检疫关员：**出现症状后第二天您是否有继续工作？

Officer: Did you continue working the day after you developed the symptoms?

**大厨：**我第二天上午没有工作，但是下午好一点后就回到厨房工作了。

Chief Cook: I didn't work the next morning, but I went back to work in the kitchen after I got a little better in the afternoon.

**检疫关员：**这几天都和谁有密切接触？

Officer: Whom have you had close contact with over the past few days?

**大厨：** 工作期间主要和服务员接触。做完饭后，我通常和他们在餐馆里聊天。

Chief Cook: Mostly stewards during my work. After I finish cooking, I usually chat with them in the restaurant.

**检疫关员：** 工作和交谈的过程中您是否有佩戴口罩？

Officer: Did you wear a mask during your work and the conversations?

**大厨：** 没有。直到今天早些时候，船长通知我们戴好口罩在自己的宿舱里等待检疫。

Chief Cook: No, we didn't wear a mask until the Captain told us to do so and wait in our room for quarantine earlier today.

**检疫关员：** 请给我看一下您的预防接种证（黄色本子）。

Officer: Please show me your vaccination certificate (Yellow Book).

**大厨：** 给您。我只接种过黄热病和霍乱疫苗。

Chief Cook: Here you are. I've been vaccinated against yellow fever and cholera only.

**检疫关员：** 好的，5 分钟已经到了，请给我体温计。

Officer: Okay, the five minutes are up, please give me the thermometer.

**大厨：** 给您，长官。

Chief Cook: Here you are, sir.

**检疫关员：** 目前体温 37.8℃，还是有发热的症状。接下来，您将接受必要的医学检查。请配合我们。

Officer: It's 37.8℃ and you still have fever symptoms. Next, you'll undergo some necessary medical exams. Please cooperate with us.

**大厨：** 好的。

Chief Cook: Sure.

**检疫关员：**（咽部检查）请您微微后仰头部，张开嘴，并说“啊……”。

Officer: (Pharynx examination) Please tilt your head back slightly, open your mouth, and say “ah...”.

（肺部检查）请放松。轻微张口，做均匀平静呼吸。做深呼吸 / 屏气 / 咳嗽。

(Lung examination) Please relax. Open your mouth slightly and breathe steadily and calmly. Take a deep breath/hold your breath/cough.

（腹部检查）请平躺，全身放松，双手置于身体两侧，两腿屈曲稍分开，张口缓慢腹式呼吸。

(Abdominal examination) Please lie on your back, relax your body from head to toe, put your hands on your sides, bend your knees with your legs slightly apart, open your mouth and breathe slowly from your belly.

**大厨：**我的身体有什么异常吗？

Chief Cook: Do I have any abnormal physical condition?

**检疫关员：**暂时没有发现任何异常。

Officer: No thing abnormal has been found so far.

**大厨：**我就只是感觉有些发热和疲惫。

Chief Cook: I only feel feverish and tired.

**检疫关员：**我们需要进行咽拭子和血液样本的采集。这是采样知情同意书。请仔细阅读相关内容后再签字。请积极配合我们的工作。

Officer: We're going to take a throat swab and a blood sample. Here's the form of Informed Consent for Sampling. Please read it carefully before you sign. We appr-eciate your cooperation in this.

**大厨：**没问题。我会配合好。

Chief Cook: No problem. I'll cooperate with you.

**检疫关员：**（采集咽拭子样本）我们现在要进行咽拭子样本的采集。请您微仰头部，张大嘴，并说“啊……”。好了，采集完毕。

Officer: (Taking a throat swab) We're taking a throat swab. Please tilt your head back slightly, open your mouth, and say "ah...". Okay, we're done.

（采集血液样本）现在要进行静脉血样本的采集，请您充分暴露手臂，我们将采集静脉血液。
(Taking a blood sample) We're going to take a venous blood sample. Please fully expose your arm for a venous draw.

**检疫关员：**好了，样品都已经采集完成。请您在宿舱内等待，做好个人防护。如果有出现其他症状请及时报告给船长。谢谢您的配合。
Officer: Okay, we're done. Please wait in your room and maintain good personal protection. If you develop any other symptoms, please notify the captain immediately. Thank you for your cooperation.

**大厨：**谢谢，麻烦你们了。我会配合好的。
Chief Cook: Thank you for the trouble you've taken. I'll cooperate with you.

**（完成其余 4 名船员的检疫排查工作后返回船长办公室）**
(Returning to the Captain's Office after completing the screening of the other four crew members)

**检疫关员：**船长，体温检测结果显示 5 名船员仍然有发热的情况。我们的同事已经采集这 5 名船员的咽拭子和血液样本。我们将把样本拿去医学实验室做相关的检验，才能最终确定是否由传染病引起发热。
Officer: Captain, the temperature measurement results show that the five crew members still have a fever. Our colleagues have collected throat swabs and blood samples from them. These samples will be taken to our medical lab for tests so that we can finally determine whether the fever is caused by an infectious disease.

**船长：**大概需要多长时间？
Captain: How long it will take?

**海关关员：**大约 4 小时。因此，这艘船舶仍需等候，发热的船员仍需隔离。其他人员不得上下船舶和装卸货物。

Officer: About 4 hours. As such, the ship still needs to wait, and the feverish crew members must remain isolated. No one is allowed to leave or board this ship , and cargo loading and unloading is not permitted.

**船长：** 好的，长官。非常感谢你们。

Captain: All right , sir. Thank you very much.

**（实验室检测结果反馈）**

(Laboratory test results transmitted)

## 第五节 后续处置

## SECTION V PERFORMING FOLLOW-UP PROCEDURE

**检疫关员：** 船长，实验室检测的结果出来了，我们进行了多种传染病的排查。结果显示 5 名船员甲型流感病毒呈阳性，根据你们的流行病学调查和医学检查的结果，我们确定你们船舶上出现了聚集性感染甲型流感的情况。需要对船舶做进一步的处置。

Officer: Captain, the lab test results are out, and we've conducted screenings for various infectious diseases. The results show that five crew members are positive for influenza A Virus. Based on the results of your epidemiological investigations and medical examinations, we conclude that a cluster of Flu A infections has broken out on your ship. More measures must be taken for the ship.

**船长：** 听起来很严重。我要向船公司报告这一切。接下来需要我配合做些什么？

Captain: Sounds very serious. I must report all this to the shipowner. What shall I do next?

**检疫关员：** 接下来我们会安排专门的车辆将 5 名有症状的船员转运到地方医院进行进一步的治疗，当然首先需要取得你们的同意。

Officer: We're going to arrange for a special vehicle to transfer the five symptomatic crew members to a local hospital for further treatment, but we need to have your consent first.

**船长：**我们当然同意。

Captain: We certainly agree to this.

**检疫关员：**在将 5 名船员转运后，我们将开具检疫处理通知书，要求您对您的船舶实施终末消毒工作，以清除船舶上的感染源。

Officer: After the five crew members are transferred to the hospital, we'll issue a Notification of Inspection and Quarantine Treatment, and you're required to carry out terminal disinfection on the ship to eliminate the source of infection.

**船长：**那我是否可以委托专业的检疫处理公司来做这事？

Captain: Can I hire a professional quarantine treatment company to do this?

**检疫关员：**当然可以，但该公司处理前应当将他们的处理方案交由我们审核。我们也将对处理过程进行全程的监督和效果的评价工作，以确保处理工作的效果。

Officer: Certainly, but the company should submit their treatment plan to us for review before doing the work. We'll supervise the whole treatment process and evaluate the result to ensure the disinfection is effective.

**船长：**你们真是太严谨和专业了。

Captain: You're so rigorous and professional !

**检疫关员：**谢谢您的肯定。同时，请做好其他船员的体温检测和健康监测工作，在这期间如果有出现新的船员有类似的症状，请第一时间报告给我们。

Officer: Thank you for your compliments. At the same time, please continue to check the temperature and monitor the health status of other crew members. If any other crew members show similar symptoms, please notify us immediately.

**船长：**放心吧，我们一定会做到的。

Captain: Don't worry, and we'll do it.

**（检疫处理实施完毕）**

(Quarantine treatment completed)

## 第六节 签证和放行
## SECTION VI GRANTING CERTIFICATION AND RELEASING THE SHIP

**检疫关员：**船长，您好，我们基本上已经完成了处置工作，处理的效果也合格。这是我们签发的入境检疫证书。您可以降下检疫黄旗，安排人员上下和装卸货了。

Officer: Hello, Captain, we've basically completed our response work, and the treatment results are up to standard. Here's the Pratique that we've issued. You can take down the yellow flag, and people are now allowed to get on or off the ship and load or unload goods.

**船长：**谢谢你们。真是太高效了。在这期间，我们的船员一切正常，没有再出现类似的症状。你们的处置工作工作太有效了。

Captain: Thank you so much. You've been so efficient. Over the past days, all has been normal with our crew members, and no one has shown similar symptoms. Your response work has been so effective.

**检疫关员：**漏报信息是严重违法行为，您必须以书面的形式进行深刻检查，并在 12 小时内提交给我们。

Officer: Omissive reporting information is a serious offense, and you must make an in-depth self -criticism in writing and submit it to us within 12 hours.

**船长：**我会按照您的要求做的，请放心，我保证以后绝不会再出现类似情况，也绝不会再隐瞒任何信息。

Captain: Please rest assured that I'll fully comply with your instructions, and I promise that we won't let it happen again and will never conceal any information again.

**检疫关员：** 希望以后您能尽最大努力保障好船员的健康，对航行负责，防止船员染上传染病并把传染病带到其他国家（地区）。

Officer: I hope that you'll do your best to ensure a fit and healthy crew, take responsibility for the voyage, and prevent the crew from getting infected and spr-eading the disease to any other country (region).

**船长：** 我会做好我的工作。非常感谢你们保护了我的船员的健康。

Captain: I'll do my job. Thank you very much for safeguarding my crew's health.

**检疫关员：** 不用谢。这是我的职责。我要下船了，下次见。

Officer: You're welcome. It's my job. I'm leaving the ship. See you next time.

**船长：** 下次见。拜拜！

Captain: See you next time. Goodbye!

**检疫关员：** 拜拜！

Officer: Goodbye!

# 第二部分　邮轮消化道疾病聚集性暴发事件应急处置

## PART II　RESPONDING TO THE OUTBREAK OF A CLUSTER OF GASTROINTESTINAL INFECTIONS ON A CRUISE SHIP

XX 年 X 月 X 日中午，厦门邮轮港海关邮轮旅检科接到代理报告，一艘由 K 岛开往厦门的巴拿马籍邮轮上有 20 多人出现腹泻等消化道疾病症状。该邮轮搭载 250 名船员、750 名旅客。邮轮旅检科立即核实相关信息并逐级汇报，同时指导船方做好先期处置。厦门邮轮港海关立即启动应急处置预案，准备好个人防护、流行病学调查、医学排查、样本采集、检疫处理监管等设施设备及相关单证等。当日 18 时，该邮轮靠泊厦门国际邮轮中心，海关关员立即登临开展应急处置工作。

At noon on ________, the Cruise Inspection Section of Xiamen Cruise Port Customs received a tip-off from a shipping agent that more than 20 people on a Panamanian cruise ship bound for Xiamen from Island K, had symptoms of gastrointestinal diseases such as diarrhea. The cruise ship had 250 crew members and 750 passengers onboard. The Cruise Inspection Section sprang into action, verifying the information and notifying higher officials while directing the ship to carry out preliminary treatment. Xiamen Cruise Port Customs immediately activated an emergency response plan and readied facilities and equipment and related documentation for personal protection, epidemiological investigation, medical screening, sample collection, quarantine treatment supervision and so on. At 6 pm on that day, the cruise ship docked at Xiamen International Cruise Center, and Customs Officers immediately boarded the ship for emergency response.

## 第一节 召开应急处置会议
## SECTION I HOLDING AN EMERGENCY RESPONSE MEETING

**检疫关员：** 船长、各位邮轮上的主管，你们好，我们是中国海关关员。由于你们邮轮在抵港前申报有 3 名船员、20 名旅客陆续出现呕吐、腹泻等症状，为了保护好船上人员健康，我们要对你们的船舶实施登临检疫做进一步的排查和处置工作。

Officer: Hello, Captain and all supervisors onboard, we're officers of China Customs. Since you declared before arriving at the port that three crew members and twenty passengers had symptoms like vomiting and diarrhea, to ensure the health of all people onboard, we need to inspect your ship for further screening and response.

**船长：** 感谢各位海关关员今晚如此迅速地上船调查处置。我们刚刚又接到报告有新增腹泻人员。我们迫切需要专业力量帮助我们找到原因，做好防控，防止事态进一步恶化。

Captain: Officers, thank you for coming so quickly this evening for investigation and response. We've just received a report that there're some more cases of diarrhea. We badly need professional help to find out the cause, implement proper control, and prevent the situation from getting worse.

**检疫关员：** 请介绍下该邮轮航线的基本情况。

Officer: Please tell us the ship's route.

**船长：** 我们的邮轮正在环球航行，将在厦门港靠泊两天一夜。船上有船员 250 名、旅客 750 名。上一港为 K 岛。我们从前天晚上 6：00 开始开往厦门。

Captain: Our ship is on a voyage round the world and will berth at Xiamen Port for two days and one night. We have 250 crew members and 750 passengers onboard. The last port we called at was Island K. We left for Xiamen at 6 o'clock the night before.

**检疫关员：** 您什么时候开始收到报告有人员出现消化道疾病症状的，船上有多少人有这些症状呢？

Officer: When did you start receiving reports that people onboard had the symptoms of gastrointestinal infections, and how many people onboard have the symptoms?

**副船长：** 从昨天晚上 8：00 开始，陆续有船员、旅客因为出现腹泻等症状到医务室就诊。截至目前，已经有 5 名船员、30 名旅客出现腹泻的症状。

Assistant Captain: From 8 pm yesterday, we had crew members and passengers coming to the hospital for treatment of diarrhea and other symptoms. So far, five crew members and 30 passengers have shown symptoms of diarrhea.

**检疫关员：** 船上已经采取了哪些处置措施呢？

Officer: What measures have been taken onboard?

**副船长：** 根据你们的指导，我们已经将有症状人员隔离在宿舱，取消船上聚集性活动，通过广播让新出现症状人员及时拨打医务室电话。此外，我们还将可疑食品进行封存、留样，做好公共场所随时消毒等处置措施。根据你们的要求，我们已经把过去 1 周的食谱整理出来。

Assistant Captain: As per your instructions, we've isolated the symptomatic persons in their rooms, canceled all planned group events onboard, and asked newly infected persons to call the hospital immediately through the intercom. Moreover, we've placed suspect food in sealed containers and taken samples, and disinfected the public spaces. As per your request, we've prepared a copy of the recipes that we've used over the past week.

**检疫关员：** 您目前初步怀疑可能引起该事件的风险因素有哪些？

Officer: What's your initial conclusion about the possible risk factors of the incident?

**副船长：** 每年，全球都会有一些邮轮出现消化道疾病暴发的情况。在大多数情况下，它们是由食物或饮用水中的病毒或细菌引起的。我们正在排查可能引起该事件的高风险食物及水。

Assistant Captain: Every year around the world, there're outbreaks of gastrointestinal infections on some cruise ships. In most cases, they're caused by viruses or bacteria in the food or drinking water. We're looking into the high-risk food and water that might have caused the incident.

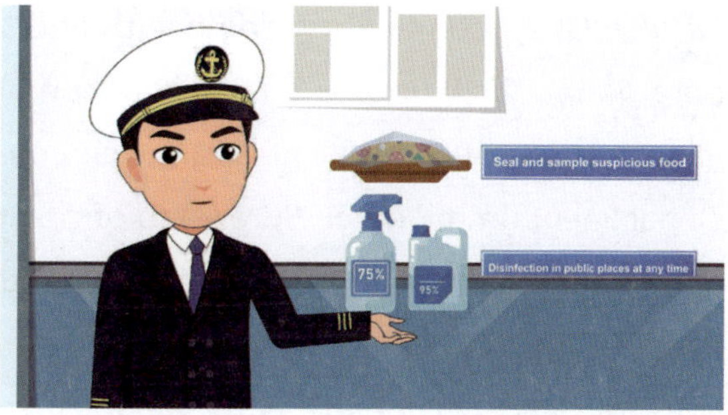


**检疫关员：**为了做好应急处置工作，我们选派了专业人员组成的不同的专业小组上船处置。船长，您可以指定一名专职人员协助，一起处理好此次事件。

Officer: As part of the emergency response to the incident, we've sent various professional teams onboard for actions. Captain, you can appoint a dedicated person to assist each of our teams in handling the incident.

**船长：**好的，我把船上的主管都叫过来了。副船长负责组织协调。你们有什么需求就和副船长说，他会安排相应的主管和你们对接。

Captain: Okay, I've brought all the supervisors here. The Assistant Captain is responsible for organizing and coordinating the actions. Just tell him what you need, and he'll ask the supervisors to assist your teams.

**船医：**不好意思，有个紧急情况，我打断一下。就诊的病人中有 1 名 65 岁的老人胃肠炎症状较重，刚刚血压下降比较厉害。他患有冠心病，目前正在医务室由护士负责照顾。考虑到船上的医疗条件有限，他申请紧急下船就医。

Ship Doctor: I'm sorry to interrupt, but we've got an emergency. Of the patients under treatment, a 65-year-old man with severe gastroenteritis has just experienced a sharp blood pressure drop. He has a coronary heart disease, and he's now being attended to by nurses in the hospital. Considering the limited medical resources onboard, he requests to leave the ship for emergency medical treatment.

**检疫关员：**好的，请放心。船员和旅客的生命健康至关重要。我们将为重症的患者开辟紧急救助的“绿色通道”。我的同事会立即联系边检部门（移民局）在船边为这位老人办理入境手续，并通知急救系统将他送往指定的医院进行抢救。您可以将他的相关证件准备好，我的同事将协同岸上的工作人员做好急救工作。下面，我们将立即分组开展处置。

Officer: Okay, don't worry. The health and safety of the crew and passengers is paramount. We'll open a "green channel" of emergency assistance for patients in severe condition. My colleagues will immediately contact the Border Control Department (Immigration Bureau) to complete the entry formalities for the elderly gentleman by the shipside and call an ambulance to send him to the designated hospital for emergency treatment. You can get his documents ready, and my colleagues will cooperate with the staff onshore to provide first aid. Next, our teams will act right away.

## 第二节 医务室信息的调查

## SECTION II OBTAINING INFORMATION IN THE HOSPITAL

**检疫关员：** 船医，您好，我们需要查阅下医疗日志。

Officer: Hello , Doctor, we need to check the Medical Logbook.

**船医：** 好的，这是电子档的医疗日志，里面详细记录了就医人员的基本信息，包括发病时间、症状、用药情况。根据你们的要求，护士准备了一份文件，里面包括近一周内有消化道疾病症状人员的基本信息。

Ship Doctor: Sure, here's the electronic Medical Logbook, which contains detailed information about the patients, including the onset time, symptoms and medication. As per your request, the nurses have prepared a document that includes the basic information about the people who have developed symptoms of a gastrointestinal disease over the past week.

**检疫关员：** 好的。根据你们的医疗日志，出现症状人员仅有个别出现低烧，大多数人是抱怨拉肚子。昨天上午 8：30 有 1 名船员因为肚子痛到医务室就医，对吗？

Officer: Great. According to the Medical Logbook, only a few of the symptomatic persons have a low fever, and most of them complain of diarrhea. A crew member came to the hospital for stomachache at 8:30 am yesterday, right?

**船医：**是的，他是酒吧服务员。当时来时只是说肚子痛，没有其他症状。我给他开了些药后，直到昨天晚上又打电话说肚子痛。

Ship Doctor: Yes, he's a bartender. He came complaining of a stomachache but had no other symptoms. I gave him some medicines, and he called again last night , complaining that the stomachache had struck again.

**检疫关员：**他有被隔离在宿舱吗？什么时候开始隔离的？

Officer: Is he isolated in his room? When did the isolation begin?

**船医：**昨天晚上因为拉肚子来就医的人多起来后，我意识到事态有点严重。在报告副船长后，开始通知有症状人员隔离在宿舱。

Ship Doctor: Last night, as more and more people came complaining of diarrhea, I realized it was a serious situation. After notifying the Assistant Captain, I had the symptomatic people isolated in their rooms.

**检疫关员：**允许服务人员和其他消化道症状人员带病上岗或与其他人密切接触而不是将他们隔离，将带来很大的风险隐患。这也违反了你们的卫生管理制度。

Officer: It's very risky to allow the bartender and others with symptoms of gastrointestinal diseases to keep working or have close contact with others instead of isolating them. This also violates your health management rules.

**船医：**是的。我们确实大意了。

Ship Doctor: You're right. We were so careless.

**检疫关员：**出现症状的其他 4 个船员中，有 1 名也是酒吧服务员，2 名是清洁工，另外 1 名是娱乐主持人。他们都住在 4 层。30 名有症状的旅客住在 8 层、9 层、10 层。旅客里有一家人同时出现腹泻的吗？

Officer: Of the other four symptomatic crew members, one is also a bartender, two are cleaners, and another one is an entertainment host. All of them live on Deck 4. The 30 symptomatic passengers live on Decks 8, 9 and 10. Do you have entire families complaining of diarrhea at the same time?

**船医：**有的。有四五个家庭昨天夜里开始出现腹泻。他们都带着小朋友。他们好像来自同一个旅行团。昨天医务室都忙不过来了。

Ship Doctor: Yes. Four or five families started having diarrhea last night. They all have children with them. It seems they're from the same tour group. The hospital was overwhelmed yesterday.

**检疫关员：**好的。船上多少比例的人员出现消化道疾病，你们会定义为感染的暴发？

Officer: I see. What's the ratio of people onboard struck by a gastrointestinal disease that would constitute an outbreak of inflection?

**船医：**这个，像这么多人，我认为感染已经发生了！我之前是在岸上的医院工作，这是我第一次在邮轮上工作，所以还不能给出一个具体的比例。

Ship Doctor: Well, with so many people infected, I think an outbreak of infection has already taken place! I used to work in a hospital on land, and this is my first job on a cruise ship , so I can't give a specific ratio.

**检疫关员：**邮轮搭载船员、旅客众多。在人群密集的环境中，呼吸道或消化道等传染病群体性暴发的风险非常大。作为一名船医，您应该熟悉邮轮上传染病暴发的定义及处置流程。

Officer: The cruise ship has so many crew members and passengers onboard. In such a crowded environment, there's an extremely high risk of a cluster of infections breaking out due to the spread of an infectious disease, such as a respiratory or gastrointestinal disease. As a ship doctor, you're supposed to be familiar with the definition of an outbreak of infection, as well as the response procedure on a cruise ship.

**船医：**是的，我刚被任命为船医不久，还需要加强学习邮轮上群体性传染病暴发的处置。

Ship Doctor: You're right, but I was appointed the ship's doctor only a short time ago, and I'm still learning how to deal with the outbreak of a cluster of inflections onboard.

**检疫关员：** 船上的船员是否都接种了霍乱等疫苗？

Officer: Have all the crew members onboard been vaccinated against cholera and other diseases?

**船医：** 是的，都有。根据公司的规定，船员都会接种黄热疫苗、霍乱疫苗、麻腮风疫苗。食品从业人员还会接种甲肝、伤寒等疫苗。

Ship Doctor: Yes, they've. Under my company's regulations, crew members must be vaccinated against yellow fever, cholera and MMR. Food workers are also vaccinated against hepatitis A, typhoid and other diseases.

**检疫关员：** 船上是否配备诺如、霍乱等消化道疾病快速检测试剂及仪器？是否开展了相关检测？请让我们看下检测试剂。

Officer: Do you have any rapid testing reagents and instruments onboard for gastrointestinal diseases, such as norovirus and cholera? Whether tests have been carried out? Would you please show us the testing reagents?

**船医：** 船上配备了诺如、霍乱快速检测试剂盒。我们已经收集了 3 名船员、10 名旅客的粪便样本。因为新增病例不断出现，我们还没来得及开展相关检测。这是诺如和霍乱检测试剂盒。

Ship Doctor: There're rapid testing kits onboard for norovirus and cholera. We've taken stool samples from 3 crew members and 10 passengers. New cases keep emerging and we barely have time for tests. Here're the testing kits for norovirus and cholera.

**检疫关员：** 这批霍乱检测试剂盒已经过期。医务室还没购买新的检测试剂盒吗？

Officer: The cholera testing kits in this batch are already past their expiry date. Haven't new ones been purchased for the hospital?

**船医：** 这个，我之前还真没有注意到。单纯发现一两个病例一般也没有用到快速检测试剂。

Ship Doctor: Um, I haven't noticed that. We rarely use testing kits when only one or two cases are reported.

**检疫关员：** 快速检测试剂过期应及时处理并购置新的检测试剂。另外，船上大肠菌群等水质微生物方面的检测是在医务室做吗？请让我们看下近期的检测记录。

Officer: You're supposed to dispose of expired rapid testing kits and buy new ones in a timely manner. One more thing, do you conduct water quality tests for microorganisms such as coliforms in the hospital? Please show us the recent test records.

**船医：** 是的，机舱部的船员会定期把水舱、厨房、宿舱等几个点的水样取好送到医务室。护士会做菌落总数、大肠菌群等检测。这是近一个月的检测记录，结果均为阴性。

Ship Doctor: Yes, the crew members in the engine room regularly take samples from the water tank, the kitchen and the crew rooms, and bring them to the hospital for tests. The nurses can carry out tests for total bacterial count and coliforms. Here're the test records for the past month, and the test results are all negative.

**检疫关员：** 好的。我们将对有症状人员开展流行病学调查、医学检查，对有症状还未留样人员及食品从业人员采集样本。在此期间，您可以对已留样样本开展诸如病毒快速检测，并第一时间告知我们检测结果。

Officer: Good. We're going to start epidemiological investigations and medical examinations on symptomatic persons, and take samples from those whose samples haven't been taken, as well as from the food workers. While we're doing the work, you can do norovirus rapid testing on the collected samples and inform us of the results as quickly as possible.

**船医：** 好的。您从哪个房间开始？

Ship Doctor: Sure. Which room will you start with?

**检疫关员：** 我们将分组按照不同舱层开展。我们先到第一个出现症状的酒吧服务员那间吧！

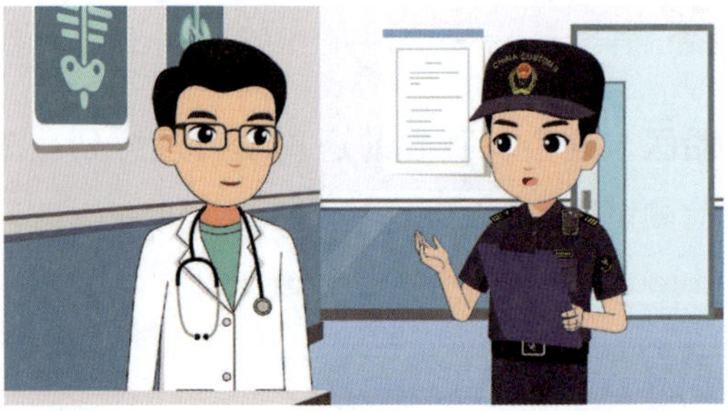

Officer: We're going to split up into multiple teams for different decks. We'll start with the room of the bartender who was the first to show the symptoms.

## 第三节 有症状人员的调查
## SECTION III INVESTIGATING SYMPTOMATIC PERSONS

### 场景一 发病船员的调查
### SCENE 1: INVESTIGATING SICK CREW MEMBERS

**检疫关员：** 您好，我们是中国海关关员，需要对您的病情做进一步的了解。请您配合。

Officer: Hello, we're officers of China Customs, we need to know more about your condition. Please cooperate with us.

**发病船员：** 好的。

Sick Crew Member: Sure.

**检疫关员：** 请提供您的护照，并告知我您的姓名、出生年月、国籍、船上的岗位和上船时间。

Officer: Please show us your passport, and tell us your name, date of birth, nationality, job title on the ship and time of boarding.

**检疫关员：** 我将为您测下体温，现在人感觉如何？还有拉肚子的症状吗？

Officer: I'm going to take your temperature. How do you feel now? Do you still have loose bowels?

**发病船员：** 现在浑身感觉没有力气，也没什么胃口。刚还拉了 1 次肚子。

Sick Crew Member: I feel weak all over and have no appetite. I've just had a bowel movement.

**检疫关员：** 好的，您的体温 36.5℃。请问什么时候开始感觉不舒服的？

Officer: Okay, your temperature is 36.5℃. When did you begin feeling unwell?

**发病船员：**昨天早上 7 点左右感觉肚子疼，后面疼得实在难受就到医务室开药了。吃完药后，我感觉好一些了。昨天中午开始拉肚子，在宿舱休息几个小时后，昨天晚上感觉好了些。昨天上晚班一会儿后又开始肚子疼，有要拉肚子的感觉。我打电话给医务室，医生让我在宿舱隔离。后面医生来看了下，继续开了口服补液盐，不过吃了感觉没什么用。

Sick Crew Member: I felt stomach pain at about 7:00 am yesterday, so I went to the hospital for medicines when the pain became unbearable. After taking the medicines, I felt a little bit better. I started having diarrhea at noon yesterday, and I felt better last night after resting for hours in the room. Yesterday, after I had been on the night shift for a while, the stomachache struck again, and I had an urgent feeling that I needed to have a bowel movement. I called the hospital, and the doctor asked me to stay in my cabin. Later, the doctor came to check on me and gave me oral rehydration salts, but I didn't think they worked.

**检疫关员：**拉得严重吗？是黏稠的，还是水样的或是其他性质的？还记得是什么颜色吗？

Officer: Did you have severe diarrhea? Was your stool sticky, liquid or something else? Do you still remember its color?

**发病船员：**它是黄黄的，非常稀。感觉是一泻千里。

Sick Crew Member: It was yellow and extremely loose and watery. The poop just shot out of my body.

**检疫关员：**除了肚子痛、拉肚子，有呕吐、肌肉痛等其他症状吗？

Officer: Do you have other symptoms such as vomiting, muscle pain... besides stomachache and diarrhea?

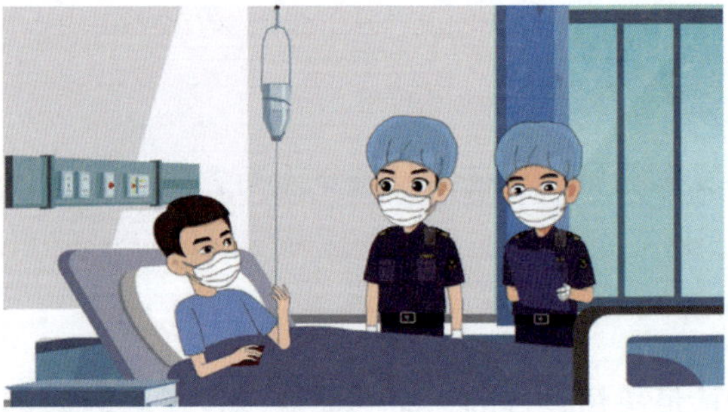

**发病船员：** 没有了。

Sick Crew Member: No, I don't.

**检疫关员：** 您个人觉得可能是什么原因导致了发病？

Officer: Do you have any idea what caused your trouble?

**发病船员：** 我觉得应该是我喝了加冰块的饮料导致的肚子不舒服！但是听广播说好多人也出现了腹泻的症状。

Sick Crew Member: I think I got an upset stomach because I had cold drinks with ice cubes! But the intercom announcement said that many people also had diarrhea symptoms.

**检疫关员：** 你在发病前几天有没有接触过什么外来的人员？他们中有人有症状吗？

Officer: Did you have close contact with non-colleagues a few days before your trouble began? Did any of them had symptoms?

**发病船员：** 我是酒吧服务员，每天都会接触来酒吧的顾客。和我一起在酒吧工作的同事昨天晚上也抱怨说出现腹泻症状，其他人就不知道了。

Sick Crew Member: I'm a bartender, and I have close contact with customers every day. My coworker in the bar also complained of diarrhea last night, but I'm not sure about the situation of other folks.

**检疫关员：** 这个是厨房提供的菜谱。请您回忆一下，出现症状前三天在哪个餐厅用过餐，把用餐情况勾选出来。

Officer: Here're the menus from the kitchen. Please try to recall which restaurants you used in the three days before you developed the symptoms, and tick the food items that you ate.

**发病船员：** 要出现症状前三天内的啊！恐怕记不全，我只能尽量回忆了。

Sick Crew Member: Three days before I had symptoms! I don't think I can remember everything, but I'll try my best.

**检疫关员：**酒吧是不是经常会举行活动？

Officer: Are events held in the bar often?

**发病船员：**船员们一般在周末会举行小型派对。对了，前天晚上有个旅行团里有人生日，举行了个生日派对。大概有 30 人参加，他们坐了三大桌。听另一个酒吧服务员说在医务室碰到那个“寿星”了，还打趣说真是有缘啊。

Sick Crew Member: The crew usually have small parties on weekends. By the way, a member of a tour group had a birthday party the night before. About 30 people joined the party, sitting at three tables. Another bartender said he ran into the birthday guy in the hospital, he exclaimed what a funny coincidence it was.

**检疫关员：**好的，派对时他们都点了些什么吃的、喝的？

Officer: Okay. What food and drinks did they order for the party?

**发病船员：**他们点了一些水果拼盘、酱牛肉、烤肠、花生、腰果、酒水和饮料。酒水和饮料都是罐装的。对了，他们还提前订了 3 个草莓蛋糕，在聚会上，甚至也给我们服务员各切了 1 块。

Sick Crew Member: They ordered some fruit platters, sauced beef, sausages, peanuts, cashews, alcoholicand non-alcoholic drinks. The drinks were canned. By the way, they also ordered three strawberry cakes in advance, and at the party, they even gave a slice of the cake to each one of us bartenders.

**检疫关员：**水果拼盘里主要是哪些水果？

Officer: What was on the fruit platters?

**发病船员：**有橙子、猕猴桃、苹果和香蕉，都是些常见的水果。

Sick Crew Member: Common fruits — oranges, kiwis, apples and bananas.

**检疫关员：**他们的酒水、饮料里有加冰块吗？

Officer: Were the drinks served with ice cubes?

**发病船员：**有四五个人喝了可乐，他们有加冰块。

Sick Crew Member: Four or five of them had coke with ice cubes.

**检疫关员：** 您在工作的过程中是否有佩戴口罩、手套？

Officer: Do you wear a mask and gloves while you were working?

**发病船员：** 口罩有戴，手套没有，戴上手套工作很不方便。

Sick Crew Member: I wore a mask but not gloves because they make me clumsy.

**检疫关员：** 好的，接下来将对您进行必要的医学检查。请配合。

Officer: Okay. Next, we're going to conduct necessary medical exams on you. Please cooperate with us.

**发病船员：** 好的。

Sick Crew Member: Sure.

**检疫关员：**（腹部检查）请平躺，全身放松，双手置于身体两侧，两腿屈曲稍分开，张口缓慢腹式呼吸。

Officer: (Abdominal examination) Please lie on your back, relax your body from head to toe, put your hands on your sides, bend your knees with your legs slightly apart, open your mouth and breathe slowly from your belly.

**发病船员：** 我身体有什么特别的异常吗？

Sick Crew Member: Do I have any abnormal physical condition?

**检疫关员：** 暂时没有发现什么异常的体征。由于您还未留存粪便等相关样本，为了快速排查发病的原因，助您早日恢复健康，现在我们需要进行肛拭子的采集。这是采样知情同意书。请仔细阅读相关内容后签名，并积极配合我们的工作。

Officer: Nothing abnormal has been found so far. Since we don't have your stool and other samples, we need to take an anal swab from you to quickly determine the cause of your infection so that you can recover as fast as possible. Here's the form of Informed Consent for Sampling. Please read it carefully before you sign. We appreciate your cooperation in this.

**发病船员：** 没问题。我会配合好的。

Sick Crew Member: No problem. I'll cooperate with you.

**检疫关员：** 好了，样品都已经采集完成。请您在宿舱内等待，并做好个人防护。船上有洗手液吗？

Officer: Okay, we're done. Please wait in your room and maintain good personal protection. Do you have hand sanitizers onboard?

**发病船员：** 有的，护士拿给我了，有交代我们上完卫生间后要及时进行手消毒。

Sick Crew Member: Yes, the nurse gave one to me, and we were told to sanitize our hands immediately after using the bathroom.

**检疫关员：** 好的。如果有出现其他症状请及时报告给船医。谢谢您的配合。

Officer: Good. If you have other symptoms, please notify the ship doctor immediately. Thank you for your cooperation.

**发病船员：** 麻烦你们了。我会配合好。

Sick Crew Member: Thank you for the trouble you've taken. I'll cooperate with you.

## 场景二 发病旅客的调查

SCENE 2: INVESTIGATING SICK PASSENGERS

**对旅客的流调、排查、采样与船员基本相同。针对旅客再调查以下信息。**

The contact tracing, screening and sampling procedures for passengers are largely the same as those for crew. The following additional information should be collected from the passenger.

**检疫关员：** 这次邮轮出行您是家庭自主旅游还是跟团旅游？

Officer: Is your family traveling independently or as part of a tour group?

**发病旅客：** 为了方便，我们这次是跟团旅游。只是懒得去做攻略了。

Sick Passenger: We're traveling as part of a group for the sake of convenience. We're just too lazy to plan everything by ourselves.

**检疫关员：** 您的家人还有团里的其他人员有出现症状吗？

Officer: Does any member of your family or anyone else in the tour group have symptoms?

**发病旅客：**我们一家四口都拉肚子了。这个旅行团有个微信群，不少人都在群里抱怨说上吐下泻。他们说他们被隔离在宿舱，感觉自己的游轮之旅都被浪费了！

Sick Passenger: All the four of us have diarrhea. The travel agency has a WeChat group for the entire tour group, and many of them complain that they've vomited and had loose bowels. They say that they felt their cruise tour has been wasted as they're isolated in their rooms!

**检疫关员：**你们旅行团在旅游期间有下船在岸上吃喝过什么吗？

Officer: What did the tour group eat or drink while onshore during the cruise?

**发病旅客：**在K岛时有下船，下船后导游带着大家分开去购物了。逛了当地的商店后，我们觉得有点累，在当地一个小店尝了下拉面，喝了店里的茶水。邮轮上有免费吃的，大家一般不会在岸上大吃大喝。

Sick Passenger: We came ashore in Island K, and the tour guide arranged for us to go shopping separately. After browsing in the local stores, we felt a little bit tried, so we had ramen and tea in a small restaurant. There was free food on the cruise ship, and we rarely ate much onshore.

**检疫关员：**你们有带当地的食物上船吗？

Officer: Did you bring any local food onboard?

**发病旅客：**没有，邮轮上不允许旅客购买吃的带上去。

Sick Passenger: No , we aren't allowed to do so.

**检疫关员：**你们家有参加前天晚上旅行团的生日派对吗？

Officer: Did your family join the birthday party with the tour group the night bef-ore?

**发病旅客：**当然有啊！旅行团的人几乎都参加了。在邮轮上一起庆祝生日是一次独特的体验。邮轮公司还特意派了娱乐主持人来活跃现场气氛。

Sick Passenger: Yes, we did. Almost everyone in the tour group went to the party. A birthday party on the cruise ship is a unique experience. The cruise operator even sent an entertainment host to liven up the a tmosphere.

## 第四节 食品、饮用水等信息的调查
## SECTION IV INVESTIGATING FOOD AND POTABLE WATER

**检疫关员：** 能介绍下船上有几个厨房、几个餐厅吗？

Officer: Would you please tell me how many kitchens and restaurants you have on the ship?

**厨师长：** 船上有两个厨房，一个供旅客使用，一个供船员使用。这里有四家餐厅，包括一家主餐厅、一家船员餐厅、一家特色餐厅和一家酒吧餐厅。

Chief Cook: We have two kitchens, one for passengers and the other for crew. And there're four restaurants, including a main restaurant, a crew restaurant, a specialty restaurant and a bar restaurant.

**检疫关员：** 主餐厅及船员餐厅都提供哪些食物？

Officer: What do you serve in the main restaurant and the crew restaurant?

**厨师长：** 主餐厅是供应给旅客的，是自助餐，会供应米饭、面食等主食，鱼、虾等海鲜，鸡、鸭等肉类，还有蔬菜、水果和面包等。这些都是免费的。船员餐厅是船员吃饭的地儿，供应的食物和主餐厅差不多。

Chief Cook: The main restaurant is open to passengers. It's a cafeteria offering staple food such as rice and pasta, seafood like fish and shrimps, meat such as chicken and ducks, as well as vegetables, fruits and bread. All of them are free. The crew restaurant is where the crew dine, and the dishes served there are similar to those in the main restaurant.

**检疫关员：** 那特色餐厅和酒吧餐厅呢？

Officer: What about the specialty restaurant and the bar restaurant?

**厨师长：** 特色餐厅提供世界各地的特色风味，是需要付钱的。酒吧餐厅主要是开派对用的，主要提供一些小菜、零食、水果还有酒水。这是过去一周各个餐厅的菜单。

Chief Cook: The specialty restaurant offers special dishes from all over the world, and diners need to pay for the food. The bar restaurant is mainly used for parties, and the food provided includes some side dishes, snacks, fruits and drinks. Here are the restaurants' menus for the past week.

**检疫关员：** 好的。有哪些餐厅供的食品是有留样的？留样时间多久？

Officer: Great. Which restaurants have kept food samples? And how long are the samples kept?

**厨师长：** 主餐厅和船员餐厅都会留样，留样时间为 48 小时。

Chief Cook: We take food samples from the main restaurant and the crew restaurant, and they are kept for 48 hours.

**检疫关员：** 前天主餐厅的菜单里有干煎虾、海蛎汤，还有蔬菜沙拉等。是否有留样？

Officer: The main restaurant's menu from the day before yesterday included dry fried shrimps, oyster soups and vegetable salads , etc. Did you take samples?

**厨师长：** 蔬菜沙拉、鸡肉等有留样。海鲜平时都是供不应求，我们没有留样。

Chief Cook: We took samples of vegetable salads, chicken, etc. Seafood is usually in short supply , and we don't take samples.

**检疫关员：** 虾、海蛎等海鲜属于高风险食物，必须要留样。请带我们看下贴有时间控制标签的食品。

Officer: Seafood, like shrimps and oysters, is high-risk food whose samples must be taken. Please show us the food items labeled with time control information.

**厨师长：** 好的，我们在邮轮上制订了特殊的时间控制计划，严格遵守食品时间控制要求。标签上详细记录了食品名称、制作时间及有效期。

Chief Cook: All right. We have a special time control plan on the cruise ship and comply with strict time control requirements for food. The name of the food, the time of preparation and the expiration date are clearly marked on the label.

**检疫关员：** 这个糕点已经过有效期了，应该及时清理掉。

Officer: This pastry is already past its expiry date and should be disposed of in a timely manner.

**厨师长：** 不好意思，确实是我们工作人员的疏忽。我将会加强对他们工作的监督和管理。

Chief Cook: I'm very sorry. The workers were so careless. I promise to strengthen the supervision and management of their jobs.

**检疫关员：** 船上是如何对食品从业人员进行培训及考核的？是否有相关记录？

Officer: How are food workers onboard trained and how is their performance evaluation? Do you keep records of training and performance evaluation?

**厨师长：** 每一位上船的船员都会进行食品安全、卫生方面的基础培训。所有食品从业人员都会进行专门的卫生培训和考核。这些是相关的培训及考核记录。

Chief Cook: All crew members receive basic training in food safety and hygiene. All food workers are subjected to special hygiene training and performance evaluation. Here're the records of training and performance evaluation.

**检疫关员：** 好的。每天上岗时，您会开展食品安全方面的监督和指导吗？

Officer: Good. Do you supervise and guide the food workers on food safety at work every day?

**厨师长：** 每次上岗时，我都会检查他们是否有戴好帽子、口罩、手套等，向他们强调在工作过程中需要注意的事项。在他们工作过程中，我也会做好监督，防止食品安全事件发生。

Chief Cook: At work, I check whether they wear hats, masks and gloves. And I make clear the dos and don'ts for their jobs. I also keep a close eye on their work to prevent food safety incidents.

**检疫关员：** 船上有饮料自动售货机、制冰机吗？是否都在正常使用？

Officer: Do you have beverage dispensers and icemakers onboard? Do they work properly?

**厨师长：** 主餐厅和船员餐厅有饮料自动售货机，各个餐厅都有制冰机。但是在这个寒冷的季节，只有酒吧有用到冰块。

Chief Cook: There're beverage dispensers in the main restaurant and the crew restaurant, and icemakers in all the restaurants. But in this cold season, ice cubes are used in the bar only.

**检疫关员：** 蔬菜沙拉里都有什么蔬菜？是怎么做的？

Officer: What vegetables do you have in the salads? And how are the salads made?

**厨师长：** 有生菜、西红柿、黄瓜。我们先用清水清洗一遍，然后用消毒混合水冲洗，再用清水清洗，最后在砧板上切好、入盘。

Chief Cook: There're lettuces, tomatoes and cucumbers. We wash the vegetables with clean water first, then rinse them with disinfectant-mixed water and with clean water again, and finally cut them on a chopping board and put them on a plate.

**检疫关员：** 消毒剂的配制是专人负责吗？

Officer: Is there any one responsible for preparing the disinfectant?

**厨师长：** 是的，我手下有个专门管理洗菜的，他每天都会统一配制消毒剂。

Chief Cook: Yes, I have a subordinate who is responsible for washing vegetables, and he prepares the disinfectant every day.

**检疫关员：** 我看这个砧板上面还有一些油渍，有切过其他东西吗？

Officer: I can see some oil stains on this chopping board, did you use it for anything else?

**厨师长：** 这个砧板也会切已经煮熟、腌制好的酱牛肉。

Chief Cook: We also cut sauced beef, cooked and marinated, on it.

**检疫关员：**酱牛肉属于熟食，和蔬菜不应共用砧板。这个酱牛肉放在哪里保存？

Officer: Sauced beef is cooked food, and a chopping board isn't supposed to be used for both cooked food like sauced beef and uncooked food like vegetables. Where do you keep the sauced beef?

**厨师长：**我们把它放在冷藏暂存柜，温度一般控制在 4℃。

Chief Cook: We keep it in this temporary freezer at at emperature of about 4℃.

**检疫关员：**这个冷藏柜里怎么还有生鸡蛋？冷藏柜不应生熟混放。

Officer: Why are there raw eggs in the freezer? You aren't supposed to put raw and cooked food together in the freeze.

**厨师长：**这个……厨房里鸡蛋用得比较多。每次要用时从库房里拿太麻烦了，所以我们放了一些在这里。

Chief Cook: Um... we use a lot of eggs in the kitchen. It's too troublesome to take them out of the storage room every time we need them, so we keep some here.

**检疫关员：**好的。我们将从厨房和餐厅里保存的食物、水和饮料以及制冰机里的冰块中采集样本送实验室做针对性的致病微生物检测。采集后，请带我们到库房做进一步的调查。

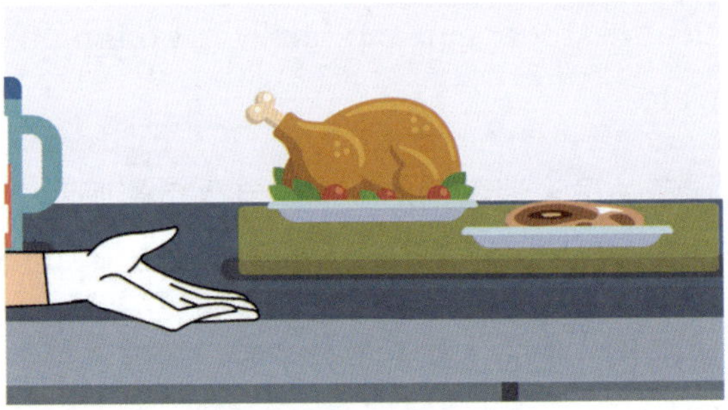

Officer: All right. We're going to collect samples from the food kept, water and drinks in the kitchen and restaurants, as well as ice cubes in the icemakers, for pathogenic microorganism tests in the lab. After we finish collecting the samples, you can take us to the food storage room for further investigation.

**厨师长：**好的。我们将积极配合。

Chief Cook: Sure. We'll fully cooperate with you.

**检疫关员：** 能提供下最近一个月库房的出入库记录吗？近期是否有新上一些食品？

Officer: Would you please show me the records of the food storage room's incoming and outgoing goods for the past month? Have you bought any new food recently?

**库房主管：** 好的。这是近一个月的出入库记录。上一周，我们在日本新上了一批牛肉，还上了一些草莓、苹果等水果，以及番茄、生菜等蔬菜。

Storage Supervisor: Okay. Here are the records for the past month. Last week, in Japan, we bought some beef, as well as some fruits such as strawberries and apples, and vegetables such as tomatoes and lettuces.

**检疫关员：** 草莓里有几颗已经发霉了。你们应该及时清理。

Officer: Some of the strawberries are moldy. You should have discarded them in a timely manner.

**库房主管：** 非常抱歉，是我们工作失误。我们将及时排查、清理腐烂的水果。

Storage Supervisor: I'm very sorry. It's our fault. We'll check the food and dispose of the rotting fruits right away.

**检疫关员：** 冻库里的肉类是拿到厨房直接加工？还是会在这边先进行加工？

Officer: Do you process the meat from the freezer directly in the kitchen? Or is the meat processed here first?

**库房主管：** 我们这里有个解冻库，可以进行初加工。肉类、鱼类的解冻有不同的区域，砧板、切刀都是有分开使用的。

Storage Supervisor: We have a thawing room here for initial processing. Frozen meat and fish are thawed separately, and separate chopping boards and knives are used.

**检疫关员：** 蔬菜、水果也会在这里先处理一下吗？

Officer: Do you process vegetables and fruits here first?

**库房主管：** 不会。蔬菜、水果一般在厨房清洗、加工。

Storage Supervisor: No. They're usually cleaned and processed right in the kitchen.

**检疫关员：**好的。根据你们的供餐情况结合流行病学调查组的调查信息，我们将对你们库房中的虾、海蛎等海鲜，生菜、番茄等蔬菜，草莓、苹果等水果采集样本，并送实验室进行检测。

Officer: Okay. Based on the information about your food service and the findings of the epidemiological investigation team, we're going to collect samples in your storage room from the seafood like shrimps and oysters, vegetables like lettuces and tomatoes, and fruits like strawberries and apples, and send them to the lab for tests.

**库房主管：**好的。我们将积极配合。

Storage Supervisor: No problem. We'll fully cooperate with you.

## 第五节 船上卫生控制措施调查

## SECTION V INVESTIGATING SANITATION CONTROL MEASURES ONBOARD

**检疫关员：**针对船上发生的消化道聚集性疾病，你们采取了卫生控制哪些卫生控制措施？

Officer: What sanitation control measures have you taken to deal with the outbreak of the cluster of gastrointestinal infections on the ship?

**环境官：**昨天夜里，当有拉肚子症状的人员陆续到医务室就医时，船医就将相关情况报告给副船长、船长。船上立即启动胃肠炎红色应急响应。一是将所有有症状的人员隔离在宿舱。二是取消了所有计划的聚集性活动。三是将相关情况告知船员及旅客，以避免引起恐慌，并要求有新症状的人员及时拨打医务室电话。四是排查食物、生活用水的风险，将生活用水的余氯调到 2ppm 以上。五是对垃圾、手可能接触的表面用 1000ppm 含氯消毒剂消毒。六是要求船上人员加强个人防护及卫生安全意识。

Environmental Officer: Last night, when people with diarrhea symptoms came to the hospital for medical treatment, the Ship Doctor notified the Assistant Captain and the Captain. A red-alert emergency response to gastroenteritis was immediately activated on the ship. First, we isolated all the symptomatic persons in their rooms. Second, we canceled all planned group events. Third, we informed the crew members and passengers to avoid causing panic, and asked all people who had also developed symptoms to call the hospital immediately. Fourth, we checked the food and drinking water for risks, and increased the residual chlorine content of drinking water to more than 2ppm. Fifth, we used disinfectant containing 1,000ppm chlorine to disinfect waste and surfaces which hands may touch. Sixth, we required everyone onboard to pay more attention to personal protection, hygiene and safety.

**检疫关员：** 根据船上的信息，有旅客出现呕吐症状。他们的呕吐物是如何处理的？

Officer: According to the ship's information, some passengers vomited. How did you dispose of the vomit?

**环境官：** 将含氯消毒剂直接喷在呕吐物上，用浸有消毒剂的抹布覆盖呕吐物，再收集进医疗垃圾袋中，送至垃圾站焚化。

Environmental Officer: We sprayed chlorine-containing disinfectant on the vomit, cover up the vomit with a rag soaked in disinfectant, scoop it up and put it into a medical waste bag, and send it to the waste station for incineration.

**检疫关员：** 有处理呕吐物的相关记录吗？

Officer: Do you keep records of vomit disposal?

**环境官：** 我们只保留不同区域的消毒记录，没有针对呕吐物的单独记录。

Environmental Officer: We only keep records of disinfection in individual areas, but no specific records of vomit disposal.

**检疫关员：** 根据你们提供的消毒记录，我们没有找到酒吧今天的消毒记录。

Officer: In the disinfection records, we can't find information about today's bar disinfection.

**环境官：** 这是我们的疏忽。负责该区域消毒的清洁工也出现症状了，我们还没安排其他人员替代他。

Environmental Officer: It's our fault. The cleaner in charge of bar disinfection has also developed symptoms, and we haven't got a replacement for him.

**检疫关员：** 请立即检测下厨房还有宿舱里生活用水的余氯含量。

Officer: Please measure the residual chlorine content of the drinking water in the kitchen and the rooms now.

**环境官：** 好的。经过检测，厨房生活用水余氯为 2.05ppm，宿舱生活用水余氯为 2.08 ppm。

Environmental Officer: Okay. We've finished that , and the residual chlorine content is 2.05 ppm and 2.08 ppm for the kitchen and the rooms, respectively.

**检疫关员：** 出现症状人员的衣物是否有用单独的洗衣设备进行清洗？

Officer: Do you have a separate washing machine for the symptomatic persons' clothes?

**环境官：** 有的，船上有 7 套洗涤设备，其中有 1 套是专供有症状人员的衣物的洗涤。控制面板中有设定专用的程序，其药剂浓度、水温都会更加严格。

Environmental Officer: Yes, there're seven washing machines onboard, one of which is used exclusively for the symptomatic persons' clothes. On the control panel, the concentration of chemicals and water temperature can be strictly programmed.

**检疫关员：** 船上的垃圾是如何处理的？

Officer: How do you dispose of the waste onboard?

**环境官：** 船上有焚烧炉，不同类型的固体垃圾分类存放、处理。有症状人员的垃圾单独收集、打包、消毒、处理。

Environmental Officer: We have an incinerator onboard, and different types of solid waste are stored and disposed of separately. The symptomatic persons' waste is collected, packed, disinfected and disposed of separately.

**检疫关员：** 污水呢？

Officer: What about the black water?

**环境官：** 船上的污水按照处理要求消毒后通过生化反应处理。同时，船上会为有症状人员配备消毒剂，以便他们可以对相关区域进行喷洒消毒及手消毒。

Environmental Officer: The waste water onboard is disinfected and then disposed of through biochemical reaction according to the treatment requirements. At the same time, disinfectant sprays and hand sanitizers are provided for the symptomatic persons to keep their rooms and hands clean.

## 第六节 后续处置

## SECTION VI PERFORMING FOLLOW-UP PROCEDURES

**检疫关员：** 经过各个应急处置小组的调查、采样和处置，样本已第一时间送至实验室，结果很快就会出来。另外，重症人员早前已通过“绿色通道”经救护车送往医院，目前正在接受治疗。

Officer: The emergency response teams have completed the investigation, sampling and treatment procedures, and the samples have been sent to the lab for tests; the results will come out soon. Meanwhile, the patient in severe condition has been rushed to hospital in an ambulance through the “green channel” , and he's currently receiving medical treatment.

**船长：** 好的。非常感谢你们连夜处置此次事件。船员和旅客完全理解你们的工作，希望能尽快找到“幕后真凶”。

Captain: Great. Thank you very much for responding to this incident overnight. The crew members and passengers fully understand your work and hope to find out the "real culprit" as soon as possible.

**检疫关员：** 我们需进一步汇总相关信息及讨论研究。现在船舶仍需等候，有症状的人员仍需隔离，其他人员不得上下船舶和装卸货物。

Officer: We need to further review and discuss all information collected. The ship still needs to wait, and the symptomatic persons should remain isolated. No one is allowed to leave or board this ship, and cargo loading and unloading is not permitted.

**船长：** 好的，我们将按照要求做好相关工作。

Captain: All right, we'll do our part as required.

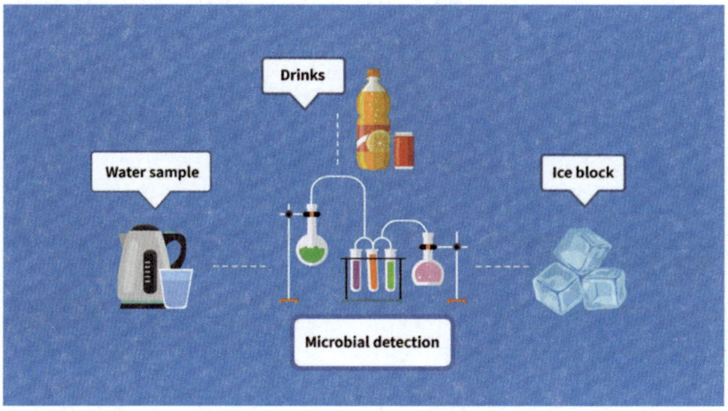


**（实验室结果反馈）**

(Laboratory test results transmitted)

**检疫关员：** 船长，实验室检测的结果出来了。我们进行了多种传染病的排查，最终在送检的人体样本及草莓中检出诺如病毒阳性。综合流行病学调查、医学检查及实验室检测结果，我们确定该邮轮上出现了聚集性感染诺如病毒的情况，需要对该邮轮做进一步的处置。

Officer: Captain, the lab test results are out. We've conducted screening for various infectious diseases and detected norovirus in the tested samples from the patients and strawberries. Based on the results of the epidemiological investigations, medical exams and lab tests, we conclude that there's a cluster of norovirus infections on your ship. More measures must be taken for the ship.

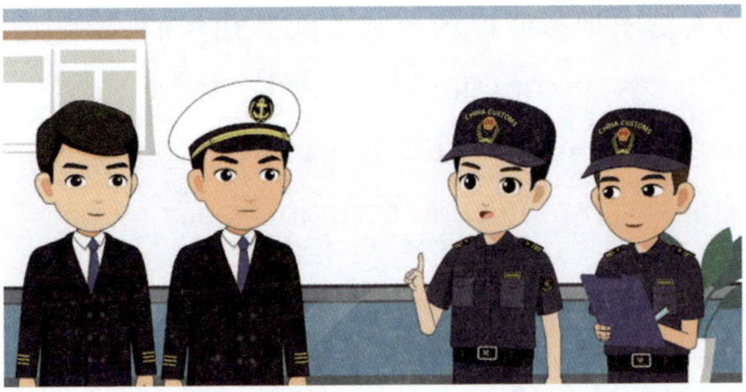

**船长：** 听起来很严重。我必须向邮轮公司报告这一情况。接下来需要我做些什么？

Captain: Sounds very serious. I must report all this to the cruise operator. What shall I do next?

**检疫关员：** 我们将开具检验检疫处理通知书，您需要对该邮轮实施终末消毒，以清除邮轮上的感染源。

Officer: We'll issue a Notification of Inspection and Quarantine Treatment, and you're required to carry out terminal disinfection on the ship to eliminate the source of infection.

**船长：** 那我是否可以委托专业的检疫处理公司来做这件事？

Captain: Can I hire a professional quarantine treatment company to do this?

**检疫关员：** 当然可以，但处理公司处理前应当将他们的处理方案交由我们审核。我们将对处理过程进行全程监督和效果评价，以确保处理工作的效果。

Officer: Certainly, but the company should submit their treatment plan to us for review before doing the work. We'll supervise the whole treatment process and evaluate the results to ensure the disinfection is effective.

**船长：** 你们真是太严谨和专业了！

Captain: How rigorous and professional you're!

**检疫关员：** 谢谢您的肯定。同时，请做好邮轮上其他人员的体温检测和健康监测工作。如果有新的人员出现类似症状，请立即通知我们。

Officer: Thank you for your compliments. At the same time, please continue to check the temperature and monitor the health status of all other people onboard. If any one shows similar symptoms, inform us immediately.

**船长：**放心吧，我们会做到的。

Captain: Sure, we'll do it.

## 第七节 签证和放行
## SECTION VII GRANTING CERTIFICATION AND RELEASING THE SHIP

**检疫关员：**船长，你好，到目前为止，所有的处置工作已告一段落，处理的效果也合格了。这是我们签发的船舶入境检疫证。您可以降下检疫黄旗，安排人员上下船和装卸货物了。

Officer: Hello, Captain, we've largely completed our response work, and the treatment results are up to standard. Here's the Pratique that we've issued. You can take down the yellow flag, and people are now allowed to get on or off the ship and load or discharge goods.

**船长：**谢谢你们。真是太高效了。在这期间邮轮上的人员一切正常，没有再出现类似的症状。你们的处置太有效了。船员和旅客可以安全放心地在厦门游玩。

Captain: Thank you so much. You've been so efficient. Over the past days, all has been normal with the people onboard, and no one has shown similar symptoms. Your response work has been so effective. The crew members and passengers can have a good time in Xiamen now without having to worry about anything.

**检疫关员：**这次聚集性诺如病毒事件的暴发暴露出邮轮上在公共卫生管理方面还是存在很多漏洞。在检查过程中已逐一点出，需要你们作出整改。

Officer: The outbreak of a cluster of norovirus infections on the ship has revealed quite a few loopholes in public health management onboard. These loopholes have all been identified during the inspection process, and you must take corrective action.

**船长：** 感谢你们对我们工作作出这么认真、细致、有针对性地指导和批评。我保证以后绝不会出现类似情况。我会及时上交整改报告。

Captain: We appreciate your elaborate and pertinent guidance and comments on our work. I promise that we'll not let it happen again. I'll submit a correction report in a timely manner.

**检疫关员：** 希望以后您能尽最大的努力提升船员公共卫生安全意识，保障好船员和旅客的健康。

Officer: I hope that going forward, you'll do your best to increase the crew's health and safety awareness and safeguard the health of the crew members and passengers.

**船长：** 我会做好相关工作。非常感谢你们及时找到致病原，保护了船员和旅客的健康。

Captain: I'll surely do that. Thank you very much for finding out the cause of the infections so quickly and protecting the health of the crew members and passengers.

**检疫关员：** 不用谢，这是我们的职责。下次见，拜拜。

Captain: You're welcome, this is our responsibility. See you next time, goodbye!

**船长：** 拜拜！

Captain: Goodbye!

# 第四章
CHAPTER IV

# 国际旅行健康服务
HEALTH SERVICES FOR INTERNATIONAL TRAVELERS

# 第一节 咨询与受理

SECTION I INFORMATION INQUIRIES AND SERVICES

## 场景一 电话咨询

SCENE 1: INQUIRIES BY PHONE

**前台工作人员：** 您好！这里是厦门国际旅行卫生保健中心（厦门海关口岸门诊部）。请问有什么能帮您？

Receptionist: Hello! this is Xiamen International Travel Healthcare Center (Xiamen Customs Port Outpatient Department). What can I do for you?

**Roberts 先生：** 您好！我是厦门 TJ 飞机维修公司国际业务部的 Roberts。近期我们公司将有一批国际员工要来厦门工作，需要到贵单位体检，我想了解你们能提供哪些服务项目。

Mr. Roberts: Hello! My name is Roberts and I'm from the International Business Department of TJ (Xiamen) Aircraft Engineering Company. We have a group of international employees coming to Xiamen. They need to undergo physical examinations with you, and I'd like to know what services you offer.

**前台工作人员：** 好的，我们中心主要服务对象就是国际旅客。我们提供广泛的国际旅行卫生保健服务，包括旅行健康咨询、健康评估、疫苗接种和健康体检。我们还能根据旅客的需要提供一些旅行卫生保健用品。

Receptionist: Well, our center caters to international travelers. We offer a wide range of healthcare services, including health information for travelers, health assessment, vaccination and physical examination. We also provide some healthcare products for travelers according to their needs.

**Roberts 先生：** 听起来真不错。那贵中心有哪些科室和专科医生呢？

Mr. Robertts: Sounds pretty good. What departments and specialists do you have?

**前台工作人员：** 我们设有内科、外科、耳鼻喉科、放射科、心电图科、B 超科、检验科和疫苗接种室等。有主任医生 7 名，医生 8 名，护理人员 10 多名。他们都有丰富的临床经验，并且都受过旅行卫生保健专业培训，擅长旅行相关疾病的预防、诊断和初步处理。

Receptionist: We have departments for internal medicine, surgery, ENT, radiology, electrocardiography, B-scan ultrasonography and laboratory tests, as well as a vaccination section. We have seven chief physicians, eight physicians and over ten nursing personnel. All of them have rich clinical experience and have received special training in travel healthcare, especially in prevention, diagnosis and preliminary treatment of travel-related illnesses.

**Roberts 先生：** 哦，您这边还能提供疫苗接种服务……您能否给我介绍一下都有哪些具体项目呢？

Mr. Roberts: Great, you also offer vaccination services... Would you please tell me what specific services are available?

**前台工作人员：** 没问题。我们中心设立了疫苗接种科，专门负责这方面的工作。现在我们主要能接种黄热病、霍乱、流感、肺炎、麻疹－腮腺炎－风疹、水痘、流行脑膜炎、脊髓灰质炎、甲肝、乙肝、戊肝、人乳头瘤状病毒等十几种疫苗。

Receptionist: Sure. We have a vaccination department specializing in these services. At present, we provide vaccination for over a dozen diseases, including yellow fever, cholera, influenza, pneumonia, MMR, chickenpox, epidemic meningitis, poliomyelitis, hepatitis A, hepatitis B, hepatitis E and human papilloma virus.

**Roberts 先生：** 那能提供国际预防接种证书吗？

Mr. Roberts: Can you issue international vaccination certificates?

**前台工作人员：** 可以的。我们中心是厦门海关所属事业单位，可以签发国际通用的预防接种证书。
Receptionist: Yes. Our center is a public institution affiliated with Xiamen Customs, and we can issue internationally recognized vaccination certificates.

**Roberts 先生：** 那贵中心的员工会说英语吗？
Mr. Roberts: Do your staff speak English?

**前台工作人员：** 会的，大部分人能说英语。如果需要，我们也可以安排能讲流利英语的引导人员。
Receptionist: Yes, most of us can. When necessary, we can provide facilitators who are influent in English.

**Roberts 先生：** 那太好了。请问贵中心的工作时间？
Mr. Roberts: That's great. May I know your working hours?

**前台工作人员：** 我们工作时间是法定工作日上午 8：00~12：00，下午 2：00~5：00。
Receptionist: We work from 8 am to noon and from 2 pm to 5 pm on workdays.

**Roberts 先生：** 需要提前预约吗？
Mr. Roberts: Do I need t o make an appointment?

**前台工作人员：** 要的。您想预约哪一天呢？
Receptionist: Yes. For what date?

**Roberts 先生：** 现在我的同事们还没到齐，我想下周应该可以。无论如何，我会提前两天与您预约。贵中心的地址在哪里呢？我们可以直接坐地铁去吗？
Mr. Roberts: Not all my colleagues have arrived, but I think all of them will arrive next week. Anyway, I'll make an appointment with you two days in advance. Where is your center located? Can we go by subway?

**前台工作人员：** 我们中心位于厦门市湖里区金鼎路 31 号。附近没有地铁站，您可以乘 11 路、12 路、26 路公共汽车，在商检站下车，也可以直接乘出租车。
Receptionist: Our center is located at 31 Jinding Road, Huli District, Xiamen. There

is no subway station around. You can take Bus No. 11, 12 or 26 to the Commodity Inspection Bureau Station, or you can take a taxi.

**Roberts 先生：** 如果自行开车去，方便停车吗？
Mr. Roberts: Is there parking available if we drive there?

**前台工作人员：** 方便的，我们单位边上有一公共停车楼，停车位较为充足。
Receptionist: Yes, there is a public parking building next to our center, and there are plenty of spaces.

**Roberts 先生：** 非常感谢！
Mr. Roberts: Thank you very much.

**前台工作人员：** 不客气。这是我们应该做的。
Receptionist: You're welcome. We're glad to have been of help.

## 场景二 现场咨询

SCENE 2: ON-SITE INQUIRIES

**前台工作人员：** 您好！这里是厦门国际旅行卫生保健中心（厦门海关口岸门诊部）。请问有什么能帮助您的？
Receptionist: Hello! this is Xiamen International Travel Healthcare Center (Xiamen Customs Port Outpatient Department). What can I do for you?

**Roberts 先生：** 我是厦门 TJ 飞机维修公司的 Roberts。上周我有打过电话来咨询我公司一批国际员工来体检的事情。
Mr. Roberts: My name is Roberts and I'm from TJ (Xiamen) Aircraft Engineering Company. I made a phone call last week inquiring about physical examinations for our international employees.

**前台工作人员：** 哦，是的，我记得。那现在有什么需要吗？
Receptionist: Oh, yes, I remember that. How can I help you?

**Roberts 先生：** 我们所有的国际员工都已经到达厦门了。我们公司计划让他们这几天过来体检，今天我来商量一下具体的安排。

Mr. Roberts: All of our international employees have arrived in Xiamen. Our company plans to have them take physical examinations in the coming days, so I'm here today to discuss arrangements with you.

**前台工作人员：** 那我带您去见我们的部门主管。这边请。

Receptionist: You can see our supervisor. This way, please.

**Roberts 先生：** 好的，谢谢您。

Mr. Roberts: Great, thank you.

**前台工作人员：** 杨主任好，这位是厦门 TJ 飞机维修公司的 Roberts 先生。他来联系外籍员工来华就业体检的事情。

Receptionist: Hi, Director Yang, this is Mr. Roberts from TJ (Xiamen) Aircraft Engineering Company. He's here to arrange physical examinations for a group of expatriates.

**主管医生：** 好的。您好，Roberts 先生。请坐。

Physician in Charge: Okay. Nice to meet you, Mr. Roberts. Please take a seat.

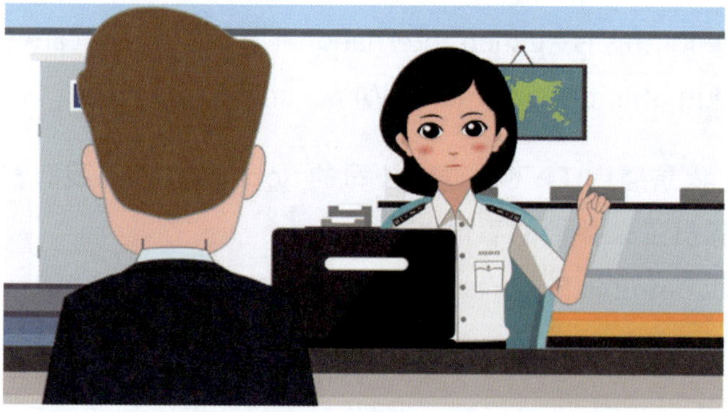

**Roberts 先生：** 杨主任好，我们公司有一批国际员工要来厦门工作一段时间。按规定他们要进行健康体检。我想知道他们近日是否可以到贵中心进行体检。

Mr. Roberts: Nice to meet you too, Director Yang. My company has a group of international employees coming to work in Xiamen. They're required to undergo physical examinations as required. I was wondering if we could book physical examinations for them with you.

**主管医生：**好的，欢迎你们的到来。他们要在厦门工作多长时间呢？

Physician in Charge: Sure, I look forward to welcoming them to our center. How long will they work in Xiamen?

**Roberts 先生：**我们这批员工一共有 25 人。他们来自美国、加拿大、英国等多个国家。根据项目安排，其中 5 人仅短期停留，预计一个月内回国；其余 20 人预计在华工作一年以上。

Mr. Roberts: There are 25 employees in this group. They're from the U.S, Canada, the U.K, etc. According to the project schedule, five of them will be working here on a short-term basis, and they're expected to return to their countries in a month; the other 20 employees will work in China for over a year.

**主管医生：**根据有关规定，拟申请来华就业、求学或定居一年以上的外籍人员须进行健康体检，体检合格后才能获得相应的签证。所以贵公司这批员工至少有 20 人应及时进行健康体检。

Physician in Charge: According to relevant regulations, foreign nationals who plan to work, study or reside in China for over a year must undergo a physical examination and will be granted a visa only after they've passed the physical examination. This means that at least twenty of these employees must take a physical examination.

**Roberts 先生：**明白。事实上为了安全起见，我们公司计划让这批员工全部参加这次体检。

Mr. Roberts: I see. In fact, our company wants all of them to take a physical examination, just to be on the safe side.

**主管医生：**好的。那他们计划什么时候来体检呢？

Physician in Charge: Sure. When will they come here?

**Roberts 先生：** 星期五早上怎么样，也就是后天？
Mr. Roberts: How about Friday morning, i. e., the day after tomorrow?

**主管医生：** 我看一下预约登记的情况……没问题，这一天预约的人数不多。
Physician in Charge: Let me check our list of appointments... No problem, we don't have many appointments for that day.

**Roberts 先生：** 太好了。那有什么需要注意的吗？
Mr. Roberts: Great. Is there anything they need to know?

**主管医生：** 是的，有几个注意事项，请让每位来体检的人员知晓：一是带上个人护照。二是不要吃早餐，保持空腹，最好是在体检前一天晚上 9 点以后不要再进食，以免影响检验结果。三是在出发国已经做过体检的，也请带上个人的健康检查资料，包括检验报告的原件，我们会根据情况进行核验。这是一份关于注意事项的小贴士，您可以带回去分发给相关人员，以便他们提前做好准备。
Physician in Charge: Yes, here are some dos and don'ts that they should know: First, they should bring their passports. Second, they shouldn't have breakfast that morning; try not to eat anything after 9 o'clock the night before the examination; otherwise, the results may not be accurate. Third, those who have taken a physical examination in the country of departure may bring their health examination documents, including the original reports, for information verification. Here are some copies of our physical examination brochure. You can hand them to your colleagues so that they can get ready beforehand.

**Roberts 先生：** 太好了，你们的服务很周到啊！那什么时候可以拿到体检结果呢？
Mr. Roberts:Excellent, how considerate you are! How soon can we get the physical examination results?

**主管医生：** 如果一切正常，下个星期一就可以拿到国际旅行健康检查证明书。但如果检查结果异常，需要进一步的检查和问询，那时间就会延迟。
Physician in Charge: If everything is fine, you'll get the "Certificates of Health

Examination for International Travelers" next Monday. But if any abnormal condition is found, further examinations and questions will be necessary. In that case, the certificate will be delayed.

**Roberts 先生：** 哦，会有哪些情况呢？

Mr. Roberts: Oh, what do you mean by abnormal condition?

**主管医生：** 例如，如果一个人的艾滋病毒检测呈阳性，我们会进一步调查。患有严重精神病、开放性肺结核以及其他严重危害公众健康的疾病的外籍人员，将被依法禁止入境。

Physician in Charge: For example, if a person tests positive for HIV, we'll perform further tests. Foreign nationals with a severe mental illness, open tuberculosis or any other disease that poses a serious threat to public health are prohibited from entering China according to the law.

**Roberts 先生：** 明白了。但愿大家都身体健康。非常感谢您的耐心介绍。

Mr. Roberts:I see. Hopefully, everyone is fine. Thank you so much for all the information.

**主管医生：** 不客气，这是我应该做的。

Physician in Charge: It's my pleasure, indeed.

**Roberts 先生：** 那我们星期五上午见。我会带我新的同事们一起过来。

Mr. Roberts: See you on Friday morning. I'll bring my new colleagues over.

**主管医生：** 好的，再见！

Physician in Charge: Good, see you then.

## 场景三 业务受理

SCENE 3: BUSINESS ACCEPTANCE

**前台工作人员：** 您好，有什么可以帮您的吗？

Receptionist: Hello, what can I do for you?

**Evans 先生：**您好，我是英国人。我要到厦门大学工作，要办理国际旅行健康检查证明书。

Mr. Evans: Hi, I'm from Britain. I'm going to teach at Xiamen University, so I need to get a "Certificate of Health Examination for International Travelers".

**前台工作人员：**好的，您近期在您的国家做过健康体检吗？

Receptionist: Okay. Have you taken a physical examination in your home country recently?

**Evans 先生：**有的。这是我最近在伦敦的体检报告原件。

Mr. Evans: Yes, I have. This is the original report of my recent physical examination in London.

**前台工作人员：**根据中国的规定，您的体检报告符合境外人员体格检查记录验证要求，我们可以直接帮您办理境外人员体格检查记录验证证明。这个证明书效果等同于国际旅行健康检查证明书。

Receptionist: Under Chinese regulations, your physical examination report is valid as a physical examination record for a foreign national, and we can issue a "Certificate of Verification for Physical Examination Record for Foreigners or Overseas Chinese". This certificate is equivalent to the "Certificate of Health Examination for International Travelers".

**Evans 先生：**这么说我不用再进行健康体检了？

Mr. Evans: Do you mean that I don't have to take a physical examination here?

**前台工作人员：**是的。请出示您的护照，并提供近 6 个月内 2 寸彩色证件照 1 张。

Receptionist: You're right. Please show me your passport and give me a 2-inch color ID photo of yourself taken within the past six months.

**Evans 先生：**好的，这是护照和照片。

Mr. Evans: Okay, here you are.

**前台工作人员：**（登记并录入系统）这是您的申请单。请核对个人信息，确认后请签字。

Receptionist: (The receptionist registers and enters the information into the system) This is your application form. Please check your personal information and sign to confirm that the information is correct.

**Evans 先生：**太好了。信息准确。（签字）

Mr. Evans: Very good. All the information is correct. (He signs on the form)

**前台工作人员：**好的。请拿好体检报告和申请单到制证室窗口领取境外人员体格检查记录验证证明。

Receptionist: Okay. Please take your physical examination report and application form to the window of the Certificate Processing Room for a "Certificate of Verification for Physical Examination Record for Foreigners or Overseas Chinese".

**Evans 先生：**好的。非常感谢。

Mr. Evans: All right. Thank you very much.

# 第二节 SECTION II 健康检查与流行病学调查 HEALTH EXAMINATION AND EPIDEMIOLOGICAL INVESTIGATION

## 场景一 体格检查

## SCENE 1: PHYSICAL EXAMINATION

### 一、内外科检查

### 1. INTERNAL MEDICINE & SURGERY EXAMINATION

**医生：**您好，请进。

Doctor: Hello , come in please.

**Davis 先生：**您好，这是我的体检单。

Mr. Davis: Hello , this is my physical examination form.

**医生：**好的，Davis 先生，这里是内外科。我们先为您测量身高和体重。

Doctor: Okay, Mr. Davis, this is the Internal Medicine & Surgery Department. We're going to measure your height and weight first.

**Davis 先生：**好的。

Mr. Davis: All right.

**医生：**请站在这台仪器上，保持立正体位……身高 180 厘米，体重 80 千克。现在请坐下，把这个体温计放在腋下，给您量一下体温。

Doctor: Please stand on this device in an upright posture... height 180cm and weight 80kg. Please sit down and put the thermometer under your armpit.

**Davis 先生：**好的，是这样吗？

Mr. Davis: Okay , is this right?

**医生：**是的，请把体温计的顶部放在腋窝的中心，紧紧夹住 5 分钟后拿出来。现在请把另一只手伸出来，我给您测血压和脉搏。

Doctor: Yes, place the tip of the thermometer in the center of your armpit, and hold your arm down tightly at your side for five minutes. Now, please extend your other hand for blood pressure and pulse measurement.

**Davis 先生：**好的。

Mr. Davis: All right.

**医生：**请卷起袖子，伸直肘部，手掌向上。

Doctor: Please roll up your sleeve, and straighten your elbow, palm up.

**Davis 先生：**我的血压是多少？

Mr. Davis: What is my blood pressure?

**医生：**135/85mmHg，在正常范围。

Doctor: 135/85mmHg, within the normal range.

**Davis 先生：** 正常的血压应该是多少呢？

Mr. Davis: What's the normal range of blood pressure?

**医生：** 正常情况下，成人收缩压低于 140mmHg，舒张压低于 90mmHg。如果收缩压高于 150mmHg 或舒张压高于 95mmHg，就要考虑是高血压了。

Doctor: For adults, normally, the systolic blood pressure is lower than 140mmHg, while the diastolic blood pressure is below 90mmHg. A systolic blood pressure over 150 mmHg, or a diastolic blood pressure over 95mmHg, suggests hypertension.

**Davis 先生：** 那还好。

Mr. Davis: I'm better than that.

**医生：** 现在我检查一下您的头部和颈部……淋巴结没有肿大，但左侧甲状腺好像有点异样。以前检查过吗？

Doctor: Now let me check your head and neck... No swollen lymph nodes, but your left thyroid gland seems to be a little different. Have you had it checked before?

**Davis 先生：** 哦，是的。过去两年 B 超检查都发现有个结节，不过医生说结节相对较小，在这两年没有变大，只需要再观察观察。

Mr. Davis: Oh, yes. B-scan ultrasonography over the past two years has showed a nodule there, but the doctor said that it's relatively small and hasn't grown bigger in the past two years, and that just more observation is needed.

**医生：** 嗯，那要注意随访。现在我需要用听诊器对您的心肺进行检查。请您将上衣的扣子解开，深吸气，再呼气。请转过身去，再作一次深呼吸……平时有什么不舒服吗？

Doctor: Well, then have periodic checks. Now I need to check your heart and lungs with a stethoscope. Please unbutton your shirt, take a deep breath, and then exhale. Please turn around, and take another deep breath... Have you had any discomfort?

**Davis 先生：** 近一个多月来时不时会咳嗽，我想可能是烟抽多了。看起来真得少抽点烟了。

Mr. Davis: I've had a cough for over a month, probably because I smoke too much. I really think I must smoke less.

**医生：**有没有发热、夜间出汗、胸部疼痛或者其他症状呢？

Doctor: Do you have fever, night sweats, chest pain or other symptoms?

**Davis 先生：**倒没有，除了天气转凉的时候。有什么问题吗？

Mr. Davis: Not really, except when the weather turns cold. Is there anything wr-ong?

**医生：**心脏还好，但肺部有听到一些啰音。我会提醒影像科医生注意检查一下，最后结合其他检查再下结论。

Doctor: Your heart is fine, but I've heard some rales in your lungs. I'll ask the radiologist to pay attention to this, and we'll make a final conclusion after reviewing the results of other examinations.

**Davis 先生：**好的。希望一切都会好起来。

Mr. Davis: Okay. I hope everything will turn out all right.

**医生：**身体和四肢都能自由活动吗？

Doctor: Can you move your body and limbs freely?

**Davis 先生：**能，我每周锻炼两次。

Mr. Davis: Yes, I work out twice a week.

**医生：**好的，那我来检查一下神经反射功能。请您面向我坐下，把左腿架在右腿上。

Doctor: Well, let me check your neural reflex. Please sit down facing me and put your left leg on your right leg.

**Davis 先生：**这叫什么检查？

Mr. Davis: What's this check?

**医生：**这是检查膝跳反射，是神经系统检查的一部分。

Doctor: This is a check of knee –jerk reflex , part of the neurological examination.

**Davis 先生：** 有什么问题吗？

Mr. Davis: Anything wrong?

**医生：** 没有问题，都很好……那我这里的检查就结束了。接下来您还需要检查眼耳鼻喉和 X 线。出门向左转并直走，看门上的指示牌可以找到对应的科室。

Doctor: Nope, all is right... I've finished my part. Next you will have EENT and X–ray examinations. Just turn left and go straight ahead, and you'll see the signs for the departments.

**Davis 先生：** 好的，谢谢您，再见。

Mr. Davis: Great, thank you, goodbye.

## 二、眼耳鼻喉检查

## 2. EENT EXAMINATIONS

**医生：** 您好，请进。

Doctor: Hello , come in please.

**Davis 先生：** 您好，医生，这是我的体检单。

Mr. Davis: Hi, doctor, this is my physical examination form.

**医生：** Davis 先生 , 这里是眼耳鼻喉检查。请坐在这里，张开口，说"啊……"

Doctor: Mr. Davis, you're taking EENT examinations. Please sit here, open your mouth and say "ah..."

**Davis 先生：** 啊……

Mr. Davis: Ah...

**医生：** 扁桃体正常，但咽喉有点充血。

Doctor: The tonsils are all right , but there is mild throat congestion.

**Davis 先生：** 哦，可能是最近烟抽得有点多吧。

Mr. Davis: Oh, maybe I've been smoking a bit too much lately.

**医生：** 吸烟有害健康，还是应该尽早戒烟。现在请把头稍微抬高一点，我要检查您的鼻子。好，没问题。现在检查眼睛，这里有几张卡片，您能看清楚上面的图片或数字吗？

Doctor: Smoking is harmful to your health, and you should quit as soon as possible. Now, please tilt your head back slightly. I'm going to check your nose. Okay, everything is fine. Time for an eye test. Here are some cards. Can you see the pictures or numbers on them?

**Davis 先生：** 这张是一只小狗，那张是数字 7，最后一张是两只蜜蜂。这是检查有没有色盲吗？

Mr. Davis: This is a puppy, that's the numeral 7, and the last one shows two bees. Is this a test for color blindness?

**医生：** 完全正确。是的，您的色觉没问题。现在测量视力。请转向右边，看着您正前方墙上的视力表。

Doctor: Exactly. Well, you have a good color vision. Now, I'm going to test your visual acuity. Please turn to the right, and look at the visual acuity chart on the wall right in front of you.

**Davis 先生：** 我看到好多的 E。

Mr. Davis: I see so many E.

**医生：** 嗯，一会儿我会从上到下指向视力表上的 E，您就依次回答我所指的 E 的开口朝向，也就是上下左右。现在先从左眼开始。

Doctor: Well, I'm going to point at the E on the chart from top to bottom, and you need to tell me the direction of the opening of the E: right, left, up or down. Let's begin with your left eye.

**Davis 先生：** 左、右、上、上、下……这个看不清楚了。

Mr. Davis: Left, right , up , up , down... I can't see this one clearly.

**医生：** 好的，换右眼。

Doctor: Okay, your right eye.

**Davis 先生：** 右、左、下、下、上……看不清楚了。

Mr. Davis: Right , left , down, down, up... I can't make it out.

**医生：** 好的，左眼视力 0.9，右眼视力 0.8。

Doctor: Okay, 0.9 for the left eye and 0.8 for the right eye.

**Davis 先生：** 哦，上一次测量都还是 1.0 呢。看来最近手机看太多了。

Mr. Davis: Oh, in my last test, it was 1.0 for both eyes. I think I've used my mobile phone too much lately.

**医生：** 还是要注意保护眼睛啊。现在检查耳朵，请跟我到隔壁的电测听室。

Doctor: You need to take good care of your eyes. Now I'm going to check your ears, please follow me to the audiometry room next door.

**Davis 先生：** 哦，这是检查听力的吗？蛮有意思的。

Mr. Davis: Oh, is this a hearing test? Quite interesting.

**医生：** 是的。请您戴上耳机，手里拿着这个按键器，每一次听到声音就按一下按键器。

Doctor: Yes. Please put on the earphones, hold this button, and press it every time you hear something.

**Davis 先生：** 好的。

Mr. Davis: All right.

**医生：** 检查好了。您的听力都正常。您可以前往下一个检查科室了。出门左转并继续向前走。

Doctor: It's all done. Your hearing is perfect. You can move on to the next department. Turn left and go straight ahead.

**Davis 先生：** 好的，非常感谢，再见。

Mr. Davis: Okay, thank you very much, goodbye.

**医生：**不客气，再见。

Doctor: You're welcome, goodbye.

## 场景二 器械检查

SCENE 2: PHYSICAL EXAMINATIONS WITH INSTRUMENTS

### 一、心电图检查

1. ECG TEST

**医生：**您好，请进。

Doctor: Hello, come in please.

**Davis 先生：**您好，医生，这是我的体检单。

Mr. Davis: Hello , doctor , this is my physical examination form.

**医生：**好的，Davis 先生，您将要做心电图检查。请躺到床上。

Doctor: Good, Mr. Davis, you're going to take an ECG test, please lie down on the bed.

**Davis 先生：**好的。

Mr. Davis: Sure.

**医生：**请卷起袖子和裤脚，衣服拉高，露出前胸。对，就这样。请放松，两手平放，自然呼吸。

Doctor: Please roll up your sleeves and trousers, and pull up your clothes to expose your chest. Yes, that's it. Relax, keep your arm flat, and breathe naturally.

**Davis 先生：**我有点紧张。

Mr. Davis: I'm a little nervous.

**医生：**放松，不要讲话。很快就检查好了。

Doctor: Just relax, and don't talk. It won't take a minute.

**Davis 先生：**我的心电图有什么问题吗？
Mr. Davis: Does my ECG show any problem?

**医生：**您的心电图有些异常变化。您之前做过心电图检查吗？
Doctor: It shows some abnormal changes. Have you ever taken an ECG test bef-ore?

**Davis 先生：**以前做过几次。
Mr. Davis: Yes, a couple of times.

**医生：**最近一次是什么时候做的？
Doctor: When was the last time you took the test?

**Davis 先生：**大概两个月以前。
Mr. Davis: About two months ago.

**医生：**您有那时的心电图报告吗？
Doctor: Do you keep that ECG report?

**Davis 先生：**有的，在这里。
Mr. Davis: Yes, here it is.

**医生：**与前次相比，这次检查几个导联上的 T 波都有显著的降低，另外早搏的次数也有明显增加。
Doctor: Compared with the last one, this test captured much lower T waves in several leads, as well as greatly increased premature beats.

**Davis 先生：**很严重吗？
Mr. Davis: Are they serious problems?

**医生：**看来是比过去加重了……医生过去给您做过什么诊断吗？
Doctor: Your heart condition seems to have got more serious... What diagnosis did the doctor make in the past?

**Davis 先生：**三年前，我的医生就认为我可能患了冠心病，但很长时间都不能确诊，直到会诊以后才确定了诊断。
Mr. Davis: Three years ago, my doctor thought that I might have coronary heart disease, but the diagnosis was not confirmed for a long time until after a consultation.

**医生：** 冠心病？
Doctor: Coronary heart disease?

**Davis 先生：** 是的，但他们说还不是很严重，所以我就出来旅游了。
Mr. Davis: Yes, but they said it was mild, so I went on a trip.

**医生：** 您平时服药吗？
Doctor: Are you on medication?

**Davis 先生：** 是的，我每天都服药。我的病情加重了吗？
Mr. Davis: Yes, I take medicines every day. Is my condition getting more serious?

**医生：** 看起来是这样的。
Doctor:It does appear that way.

**Davis 先生：** 哦，真是个坏消息……那我还能继续我的旅游吗？
Mr. Davis: Oh, that's really bad news... So, can I continue my trip?

**医生：** 您还准备上哪儿旅游呢？
Doctor: Which places are you going to visit next?

**Davis 先生：** 我原来计划下周去黄山，然后去拉萨。
Mr. Davis: I originally planned to visit the Yellow Mountains next week and then Lhasa.

**医生：** 我想目前您这情况可能不宜进行容易导致疲劳、紧张或增加心肺负担的旅行。建议您尽快到医院找专科医生做进一步检查，他们会给出对您最有利的建议。
Doctor: I don't think you are fit enough to take a trip that is tiring and tense or will put stress on your heart and lungs. I suggest you see specialists in the hospital for

further examinations as soon as possible, and they'll give you the best advice.

**Davis 先生：** 好的，谢谢您，再见。

Mr. Davis: Okay, thank you, goodbye.

**医生：** 再见。

Doctor: Goodbye.

## 二、B 超检查

2. B-ULTRASONOGRAPHY

**医生：** 是 Anderson 先生吗？

Doctor: Are you Mr. Anderson?

**Anderson 先生：** 我是。

Mr. Anderson: Yes, I'm.

**医生：** 您最近做过 B 超检查吗？

Doctor: Have you taken B-ultrasonography lately?

**Anderson 先生：** 没有。

Mr. Anderson: No , I haven't.

**医生：** 来这之前您吃过早餐了吗？

Doctor: Did you have breakfast before you came here?

**Anderson 先生：** 还没有。

Mr. Anderson: No , I didn't.

**医生：** 请脱掉鞋子，躺在诊床上，将腰带放松，衣服撩起，露出腹部。放松，自然呼吸。

Doctor: Please take off your shoes, lie down on the bed, loosen your belt , and pull up your clothes to expose your abdomen. Relax and breathe naturally.

**Anderson 先生：** 好的。

Mr. Anderson: Sure.

**医生：** 过去患过什么疾病吗？

Doctor: Have you had any disease?

**Anderson 先生：** 一年前得过肝炎，经过治疗已经好了。医生，我的肝脏有没有问题？

Mr. Anderson: I had hepatitis a year ago , but I've fully recovered after treatment. Is there anything wrong with my liver, doctor?

**医生：** 您的肝脏和脾脏都正常。您以前得过胆囊疾病吗？

Doctor: Your liver and spleen are fine. Have you had any gallbladder disease bef-ore?

**Anderson 先生：** 没有。

Mr. Anderson: No , I haven't.

**医生：** 从 B 超检查结果看，您胆囊里有少量结石。平常身体有没有不舒服？

Doctor: B-ultrasonography shows a few stones in your gallbladder. Do you feel any discomfort?

**Anderson 先生：** 没有异常。那我该怎么治疗呢？

Mr. Anderson: Not really. What shall I do?

**医生：** 目前还不需要治疗，但是要定期复查。可以了，这是您的 B 超检查报告，平常要注意饮食清淡，如果感到不舒服要及时就医。

Doctor: You don't need any treatment at this moment, but regular checkups are necessary. We're all done here. Here is your B-ultrasonography report. Remember to eat right and eat light. See a doctor if you are unwell.

**Anderson 先生：** 好的。谢谢。

Mr. Anderson: Okay. Thank you.

## 三、X 线检查

3. X -RAY EXAMINATION

**医生：** 是 Taylor 女士吗？

Doctor: Are you Ms. Taylor?

**Taylor 女士：** 我是。

Ms. Taylor: Yes, I'm.

**医生：** 请您到隔壁检查室准备 X 光检查，我会通过对讲系统与您通话。

Doctor: Please step into the examination room next door for an X-ray examination. I'll talk to you through the intercom.

**Taylor 女士：** 好的，是那个门进去吗？

Ms. Taylor: Okay, should I go through that door?

**医生：** 是的。

Doctor: Yes.

**医生：** 现在请您到角落那边的屏风处更换检查服，外套和金属饰品都要脱下来。

Doctor: Now, please change into the X-ray gown behind the screen in the corner. You need to take off your coat and remove your jewelry and all metallic objects.

**Taylor 女士：** 好的……换好了。

Ms. Taylor: Okay... I'm done.

**医生：** 现在请站在 X 光机正前方的踏板上，背部贴紧后面的靠板，肩部向前。

Doctor: Please step onto the pedal right in front of the X-ray machine, and stand there with your back against the rear plate and keep your shoulders forward.

**Taylor 女士：** 是这样吗？

Ms. Taylor: Is this right?

**医生：** 是的，请站好。我先给您拍个胸片。请保持上身挺直，深呼吸，然后屏住气。您做得很好。

Doctor: Yes, please stand still. I will take a chest X-ray first. Keep your upper body straight, take a deep breath, and then hold your breath. You're doing very well.

**Taylor 女士：**医生，拍好了吗？
Ms. Taylor: Are we done, doctor?

**医生：**好了，您可以换回自己的衣服了。记得带走您之前拿下来的金属饰品等物品。
Doctor: Yes, you can change back into your clothes. Don't forget your jewelry and other belongings.

**Taylor 女士：**拍片结果怎么样呢？
Ms. Taylor: Wha t about the results?

**医生：**有点情况。您最近咳嗽吗？
Doctor: There is a problem. Have you had a cough lately?

**Taylor 女士：**我感冒很久了，晚上咳得厉害些。
Ms. Taylor: I've had a cold for a long time, and I'm still coughing a lot at night.

**医生：**有多长时间了呢？
Doctor: How long has this been going on?

**Taylor 女士：**快一个月了……是有什么问题吗？
Ms. Taylor: Almost a month... What's the problem?

**医生：**从胸片上来看，您的左肺有一片阴影，可能是肺炎，但也不排除肺结核或其他病变。
Doctor: The chest X-ray scan shows a shadow in your left lung; it may be pneumonia, but we can't rule out the possibility of tuberculosis or other diseases.

**Taylor 女士：**是不是很严重？
Ms. Taylor: Is it serious?

**医生：**现在还很难确定。需要进一步的检查。

Doctor: At this moment , it is hard to say what it is. More examinations are needed.

**Taylor 女士：** 那要怎么办呢？

Ms. Taylor: What should I do?

**医生：** 建议您检查结束后尽快安排时间去医院找专科医生做进一步诊断。如果您需要这里的检查结果，我们可以为您拷贝一份。

Doctor: I suggest you see a specialist in the hospital for further diagnosis right after you have finished the examinations here. If you need an examination report , we can give you a copy.

**Taylor 女士：** 好的。谢谢，医生。

Ms. Taylor: Great. Thank you, doctor.

**医生：** 不客气。这是我们应该做的，也祝您早日康复。

Doctor: You're welcome. We're glad to have been of help. I wish you a quick recovery.

## 场景三 实验室检查 / 样品采集

SCENE 3: LABORATORY TESTS/SAMPLING

**护士：** 是 Brown 先生吗？

Nurse: Are you Mr. Brown?

**Brown 先生：** 是的，您好。

Mr. Brown: Yes, I'm. Nice to meet you.

**护士：** 请坐，脱去外套，卷起衣袖至胳膊肘处。

Nurse: Please have a seat, take off your jacket, and roll up your sleeves to your elbow.

**Brown 先生：** 要抽很多血吗？

Mr. Brown: Are you going to draw a lot of blood?

**护士：** 根据您检查的项目，我们需要用两个采样管采集 7mL 静脉血。这不会对您的健康有任何影响，请您放心。现在请紧握拳头。

Nurse: For all your examination items, we need two 7mL vials of venous blood. It will not affect your health in any way; don't worry. Please clench your fist.

**Brown 先生：** 好的。请问这次检查都有哪些项目呢？

Mr. Brown: Okay. What're the examination items?

**护士：** 有血常规、生化指标以及一些传染病的检测项目。现在采好了。请您拿着这根棉签按压 2 分钟左右，直到不出血为止。

Nurse: There are blood routine and biochemical indicator tests, as well as some infectious disease tests. We're done. Please press the cotton swab here for about two minutes until the bleeding stops.

**Brown 先生：** 好的。看起来不出血了。

Mr. Brown: Okay. It seems the bleeding has stopped.

**护士：** 这里还有两个小容器，请您拿着。

Nurse: Here are two small containers for you.

**Brown 先生：** 这是做什么的呢？

Mr. Brown: What are they for?

**护士：** 这是尿液采样管。请您到洗手间留取中段尿液，然后把采样管插在那边的架子上。这里有条刻度线，请注意尿量不能低于刻度线。

Nurse: They're urine sampling tubes. Please go to the bathroom and take a sample of your midstream urine with these tubes, then, place the tubes on the shelf over there. There is a scale mark here. Please be careful that the urine sample mustn't be lower than the mark.

**Brown 先生：** 好的。

Mr. Brown: All right.

**护士：** 这个是采集粪便样品用的无菌瓶。里面有个小勺，将勺子取出的粪便装进瓶子里，避免沾到水或者尿液。拧紧盖子，同样放到那边的架子上。

Nurse: Here's a sterile bottle for stool sampling. There is a small spoon in it. Use this spoon to take some stool and put it into the bottle. Be careful not to get it stained by water or urine. Screw the lid on tightly, and put the bottle on the same shelf over there.

**Brown 先生：** 好的，那所有的检查结果什么时候会出来呢？

Mr. Brown: Okay. When can I get the results?

**护士：** 一般两个工作日后。到时请您来取。

Nurse: Normally in two workdays. Come back on that date.

**Brown 先生：** 好的，谢谢。

Mr. Brown: All right, thank you.

## 场景四 证书签发

SCENE 4: CERTIFICATE ISSUANCE

### 一、签发证书

1. CERTIFICATION GRANTED

**前台工作人员：** 您好，请问您办理什么业务？

Receptionist: Hello , what can I do for you?

**Brown 先生：** 我来拿我的体检报告。上周我在这里做了体检。

Mr. Brown: I'm here to pick up my physical examination report. I took a physical examination here last week.

**前台工作人员：** 请您到大厅左边的第一个窗口找杨医生。他会向您介绍您的体检结果及有关注意事项。

Receptionist: Please see Dr. Yang at the first desk on the left side of the hall. He'll explain your physical examination results and give some advice to you as well.

**Brown 先生：** 好的，谢谢。

Mr. Brown: Okay, thanks.

**Brown 先生：** 请问是杨医生吗？

Mr. Brown: Excuse me, are you Dr. Yang?

**签证医生：** 是的，请问有什么可以帮您？

Certification Doctor: Yes, I'm. What can I do for you?

**Brown 先生：** 我是 YP 公司的 John Brown，我来拿我的体检报告。

Mr. Brown: I'm John Brown from YP Company, I'm here to pick up my physical examination report.

**签证医生：** 好的。请出示您的护照或者领取凭证。

Certification Doctor: All right. Please show me your passport or receipt.

**Brown 先生：** 这是我的护照。

Mr. Brown: Here is my passport.

**签证医生：** 您稍等。在这里。除了胆囊有个小结石，其他的都还好。

Certification Doctor: Wait a minute, please. Here is the report. Everything is fine, except that there is a small stone in your gallbladder.

**Brown 先生：** 哦，是吗？以前倒没发现。那有什么要注意的吗？

Mr. Brown: Oh, a small gallstone? I didn't know that. Is there anything I should do?

**签证医生：** 胆结石多见于爱吃高脂肪、高糖类、高胆固醇的饮品或零食的人群。我看您体形偏胖，血脂水平也接近超标了。今后还是要注意健康饮食，适当运动也会很有帮助。

Certification Doctor: People who prefer high-fat, high-sugar or high-cholesterol drinks or snacks are more likely to develop gallstones. You seem to be overweight, and your blood lipid level is almost over the limit. It is very important to eat he-althy, and moderate exercise helps, too.

**Brown 先生：** 您说得很对。看来我需要做些改变了。

Mr. Brown: You're right. I must make some changes.

**签证医生：** 这是您的国际旅行健康检查证明书。您可以到公安机关办理相关手续了。祝您在中国工作顺利，健康快乐。

Certification Doctor: Here is your "Certificate of Health Examination for International Travelers". You may complete the formalities with public security authorities. I wish you all the best working here in China.

**Brown 先生：** 非常感谢，再见。

Mr. Brown: Thank you very much, goodbye.

## 二、不予签发证书
## 2. CERTIFICATION DENIED

**Anderson 先生：** 请问是杨医生吗？

Mr. Anderson: Excuse me, are you Dr. Yang?

**签证医生：** 我是，请问有什么可以帮您？

Certification Doctor: Yes, I'm. What can I do for you?

**Anderson 先生：** 我是 TP 公司的 Anderson。昨天我接到贵中心工作人员电话，让我来拿体检报告，还说有些情况要向我了解一下。

Mr. Anderson: I'm Anderson from TP Company. Yesterday I got a call from your center, asking me to come here for my physical examination report. The caller also said that there is something he needs to ask me about.

**签证医生：** 哦，Anderson 先生……是这样的。您的体检结果有些异常，所以现在我们暂时无法为您签发国际旅行健康检查证明书。

Certification Doctor: Oh, Mr. Anderson... Here is the thing. Your physical examination results don't look totally okay, so we can't issue a "Certificate of Health Examination for International Travelers" at this moment.

**Anderson 先生：** 啊，不会吧！是什么问题呢？

Mr. Anderson: Oh, no! What's the problem?

**签证医生：** 我带您到医生办公室，我的同事会向您说明具体情况。

Certification Doctor: Please follow me to the doctor's office, and my colleague will explain it to you.

**Anderson 先生：** 哦，您不能直接跟我说吗？

Mr. Anderson: Oh, can't you just tell me?

**签证医生：** 为了保护您的隐私，我们为您安排了专科医生，一会儿他还会问您几个问题。

Certification Doctor: To protect your privacy, we've arranged for a specialist for you, and he'll ask you a few questions.

**Anderson 先生：** 看起来有点麻烦……

Mr. Anderson: It seems I'm in trouble...

**签证医生：** 您不要太紧张，请跟我往这边来。

Certification Doctor: Don't worry. This way please.

**Anderson 先生：** 好的。

Mr. Anderson: All right.

## 场景五 流行病学调查

SCENE 5: EPIDEMIOLOGICAL INVESTIGATION

**医生：** 您好，您是 Anderson 先生吗？

Doctor: Hello , are you Mr. Anderson?

**Anderson 先生：** 您好，我是 Anderson 先生。

Mr. Anderson: Yes, I'm. Nice to meet you.

**医生：** 我能问您一些个人的问题吗？

Doctor: May I ask you some personal questions?

**Anderson 先生：** 我不介意。

Mr. Anderson: Sure, go ahead please.

**医生：** 您结婚了吗？

Doctor: Are you married?

**Anderson 先生：** 没有，但我交过几个女朋友。

Mr. Anderson: No , but I've dated a couple of girls.

**医生：** 几个？

Doctor: How many girlfriends have you had?

**Anderson 先生：** 从高中到现在有 20 多个。

Mr. Anderson: I've had over 20 girlfriends since high school.

**医生：** 是否有过同性恋行为？

Doctor: Have you ever engaged in homosexual conduct?

**Anderson 先生：** 有。5 年前发生过。

Mr. Anderson: Yes, I've. It happened five years ago.

**医生：** 有过几个同性伴侣？

Doctor: How many homosexual partners have you had?

**Anderson 先生：** 至今 10 个。

Mr. Anderson: 10 so far.

**医生：** 是否用安全套等保护措施？

Doctor: Did you take protective measures, such as using condoms?

**Anderson 先生：** 有时用，有时不用。

Mr. Anderson: Some times.

**医生：** 得过性病吗？

Doctor: Have you ever been infected with any sexually transmitted diseases?

**Anderson 先生：** 得过淋病、疱疹。

Mr. Anderson: Yes, gonorrhea and herpes.

**医生：** 最近一次体检是什么时候？

Doctor: When was the last time you took a physical examination?

**Anderson 先生：** 一年前，当时没有什么问题。

Mr. Anderson: It was about a year ago , but no problem was found.

**医生：** 最近您身体有没有不舒服？

Doctor: Have you felt unwell lately?

**Anderson 先生：** 没有，很正常。我这次体检有什么问题吗？

Mr. Anderson: No. I feel well. Is there anything wrong with my results?

**医生：** 我们在您的血液样本中检出艾滋病抗体阳性。

Doctor: We've found HIV antibodies positive in your blood sample.

**Anderson 先生：** 哦，不可能吧。这不是真的。

Mr. Anderson: Oh, no. That can't be true.

**医生：** 是真的。这可能与您的性生活有关。您对艾滋病了解吗？

Doctor: It is. It may be related to your sexual life. Do you know anything about HIV?

**Anderson 先生：** 我知道，我身边有朋友就是得了这个病去世的。我不会也要死了吧？

Mr. Anderson: Yes, I do. A friend of mine has died of this disease. I'm not going to die, am I?

**医生：** 不要悲观。您现在只是艾滋病携带者。只要配合医生积极进行治疗，戒掉不良的生活习惯，您还是可以和正常人一样生活和工作。

Doctor: Cheer up. You're just an HIV carrier. You can still live and work like a normal person, as long as you follow the doctor's advice, undergo all treatments with a positive attitude, and switch to a healthy lifestyle.

**Anderson 先生：**我是不是不能留在中国了？

Mr. Anderson: Does that mean I'm not allowed to stay in China?

**医生：**您可以继续留在中国，但是我们不能为您签发国际旅行健康检查证明书。没有这个证书，您可能无法获得您的签证。

Doctor: You can stay in China, but we can't issue a "Certificate of Health Examination for International Travelers". Without this certificate, you may not be able to get a visa.

**Anderson 先生：**没有签证，我就无法在中国读书了。

Mr. Anderson: Without a visa, I can't study in China.

**医生：**很遗憾，我建议您回国后去医院做进一步检查，并尽快开始治疗。

Doctor: I'm sorry, but I suggest you take further examinations and begin treatment in the hospital right after returning to your home country.

**Anderson 先生：**也只能这样了。

Mr. Anderson: Yes, I must do that.

**医生：**这是您的体检报告。请您收好。

Doctor: Here is your physical examination report. Keep it in a safe place.

**Anderson 先生：**好的。谢谢医生。再见。

Mr. Anderson: All right. Thank you, doctor. Goodbye.

**医生：**再见。

Doctor: Goodbye.

# 第三节 疫苗接种与预防
# SECTION III VACCINATION AND PRECAUTION

## 场景一 业务咨询
## SCENE 1: INFORMATION INQUIRY

### 一、疫苗接种咨询
### 1. VACCINATION INQUIRY

**Williams 先生：** 您好，请问是杨医生吗？

Mr. Williams: Hello , are you Dr. Yang?

**杨医生：** 是的，您好！请问有什么可以帮您？

Dr. Yang: Yes, I'm. Nice to meet you. What can I do for you?

**Williams 先生：** 我是环球邮轮公司厦门办事处的经理 Robin Williams，之前有跟您电话咨询过疫苗接种的事情。这是我的名片。

Mr. Williams: I'm Robin Williams, manager of the Xiamen Office of Global Cruise Company. I made a phone call asking about vaccination the other day. Here is my business card.

**杨医生：** 哦，我想起来了。是您公司旗下邮轮船员疫苗接种的事情吧？

Dr. Yang: Oh, yes, I remember that. You were asking about vaccination for your company's cruise crew?

**Williams 先生：** 您记性真好！下周三我们公司有一艘邮轮要挂靠厦门港停靠三天。公司想为船员们安排疫苗接种。

Mr. Williams: You've got an excellent memory! Next Wednesday, we have a cruise to call at Xiamen Port for three days. We want to arrange vaccination for the crew.

**杨医生：** 好的，请问有多少船员需要接种，需要接种哪些疫苗呢？

Dr. Yang: Okay, how many crew members need vaccination, and what vaccinations do they need?

**Williams 先生：** 船上总共有 1500 多名船员，其中有 100 多名船员是两周前在新加坡换班上船的。根据我们公司邮轮卫生安全的管理要求，我们需要为这些船员安排接种黄热病和水痘疫苗。

Mr. Williams: The ship has a crew of over 1500, and more than 100 of them came onboard in Singapore two weeks ago as part of the crew change. According to our company's health and safety rules, we must vaccinate these crew members against yellow fever and chickenpox.

**杨医生：** 哦，数量可真不少。看来我们现在就得开始做准备。

Dr. Yang: Oh, you've got quite a lot of people for vaccination. It seems we must start preparing now.

**Williams 先生：** 你们现在都有哪些疫苗呢？

Mr. Williams: What vaccines do you have?

**杨医生：** 我们现有黄热病、霍乱、流感、肺炎、麻疹－腮腺炎－风疹、水痘、流行性脑膜炎、脊髓灰质炎、甲肝、乙肝、戊肝、人乳头瘤状病毒等十几种疫苗，库存数量各不一样。我看看……黄热病疫苗目前是够的，但水痘疫苗可能需要额外补充一些。

Dr. Yang: We have vaccines for over a dozen types of diseases, including yellow fever, cholera, influenza, pneumonia, MMR, chickenpox, epidemic meningitis, poliomyelitis, hepatitis A, hepatitis B, hepatitis E, human papilloma virus, etc. Their stocks vary. Let me see... We have plenty of doses of yellow fever vaccine, but we'll need more doses of chickenpox vaccine.

**Williams 先生：** 到时您能安排人员到邮轮上实施接种吗？

Mr. Williams: Can you vaccinate the crew on the cruiser?

**杨医生：** 那要看邮轮上有没有配备船医、急救药品和设施，以及供被接种人员接受医学观察的区域。

Dr. Yang: It depends on whether there are doctors, first aid supplies and facilities on the ship, and whether there is an area onboard where vaccine recipients can be placed under medical observation.

**Williams 先生**：我们的邮轮上有一个小型医院，配备有三名持证的医务人员，各类急救设备也比较齐全，应该没问题。

Mr. Williams: We have a small hospital on the cruiser, equipped with three certified medical personnel, as well as a full range of first aid supplies and facilities. Everything should be fine.

**杨医生**：好的。邮轮靠岸后我们可以先派人到现场确认一下。如果一切顺利，我们会安排专业医护人员登轮为船员接种疫苗。

Dr. Yang: Great. We'll send someone to confirm that after the cruiser docked. If all goes well, we'll send professional medical personnel to vaccinate the crew onboard.

**Williams 先生**：那太好了。

Mr. Williams: That's great.

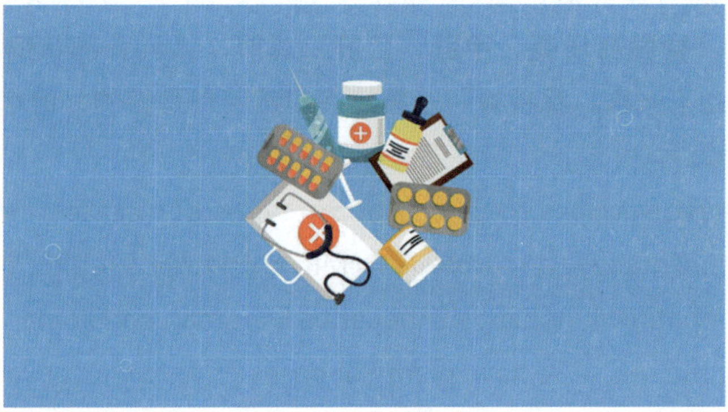

**杨医生**：我们会提前制订工作方案，包括接种的注意事项。到时可能需要船上的人员，尤其是船医为我们提供支持和配合，也请您协助提前沟通。

Dr. Yang: We'll draw up a work plan beforehand, including vaccination tips. We may need some of your people onboard, especially the ship's doctors, to assist us with the vaccination. Please talk to them about our plan beforehand.

**Williams 先生**：没问题。我们会根据您的工作方案提前做好准备。

Mr. Williams: No problem. We'll prepare for the vaccination according to your work plan.

**杨医生：**那我们保持联系。

Dr. Yang: Let's keep in touch.

**Williams 先生：**非常感谢您的悉心接洽。保持联系。再见。

Mr. Williams: Thank you very much for your time. Keep in touch. Goodbye.

## 二、预防措施咨询

## 2. PRECAUTION INQUIRIES

**Rivera 小姐：**请问是杨医生吗？

Miss Rivera: Are you Dr. Yang?

**医生：**是的。请问有什么需要帮忙的？

Doctor: Yes, I'm. What can I do for you?

**Rivera 小姐：**我公司的两位同事将要去 N 国工作一段时间。他们以前从未去过非洲。我们听说去 N 国的人必须接种疫苗，公司让我来问问有什么具体要求。

Miss Rivera: Two of my colleagues are going to work in Country N for some time. They're never been to Africa before. We've heard that travelers heading to Country N must have vaccination, so I'm here to find out the specific requirements.

**医生：**根据世界卫生组织公布的信息，N 国部分区域仍有黄热病流行，因此他们要求入境人员必须持有效的黄热病预防接种证书。

Doctor: According to information released by the World Health Organization, yellow fever is widespread in some parts of Country N, so incoming travelers are required to have a yellow fever vaccination certificate.

**Rivera 小姐：**什么是黄热病？以前好像没听过。

Miss Rivera: What is yellow fever? I don't think I've heard of it before.

**医生：**黄热病是一种由黄热病毒引起，经蚊虫叮咬传播的急性传染病，主要在非洲和南美洲部分区域流行。亚洲国家和地区没有本土病例，这可能是您之前没听说过的原因。然而，这个病比较凶险，如无免疫力的人感染黄热病，一旦发病，病死率可高达 50%。

Doctor: Yellow fever is an acute infectious disease caused by the yellow fever virus and spread to people by the bite of an infected mosquito. It is most common in certain parts of Africa and South America. No local cases have been reported in Asian countries and regions, and that is probably why you haven't heard of it before. However, it is a dangerous disease. For vulnerable people infected with yellow fever, the fatality rate can be as high as 50%.

**Rivera 小姐：** 太可怕了，那应该怎样做才不会被感染呢？
Miss Rivera: It is terrible. How shall we to prevent yellow fever?

**医生：** 接种黄热病疫苗可以有效预防这种病！我们中心可以提供黄热病疫苗接种服务，并签发国际通用的预防接种证书。
Doctor: Vaccination is an effective preventive measure against yellow fever. Our center offers yellow fever vaccination service and can issue internationally recognized vaccination certificates.

**Rivera 小姐：** 太好了……那这个证书有什么用呢？
Miss Rivera: That's great... What is the certificate for?

**医生：** 很多国家（地区）都要求有黄热病风险地区旅行史的旅客持有有效的黄热病疫苗国际预防接种证书。如果没有，在入境时可能会被拒绝。
Doctor: Many countries (regions) require a valid international certificate of vaccination for yellow fever from travelers who have been to areas exposed to yellow fever. Travelers who do not have such a certificate may be denied entry.

**Rivera 小姐：** 哦，我明白了。那去 N 国还有什么别的疫苗要打吗？
Miss Rivera: Oh, I see. Are there other vaccines that travelers heading to Country N must get?

**医生：** 在 N 国以及附近的一些国家和地区，同时有霍乱、疟疾、流行性脑膜炎等疾病流行，但也不一定都需要打疫苗。我们会根据国际旅行者的个人情况、具体行程等综合评估，建议他们采取相应的旅行卫生保健措施。

Doctor: Country N, some countries and regions nearby are also plagued by cholera, malaria, meningitis, etc., but vaccination isn't always required for these diseases. We'll evaluate the personal circumstances and specific itinerary of each international traveler and advise him on precautions accordingly.

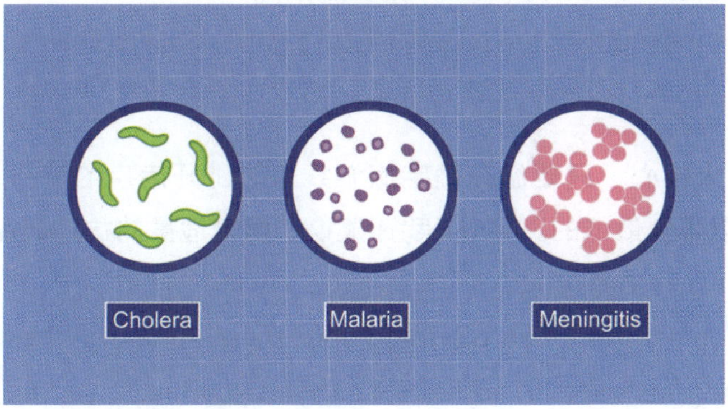


**Rivera 小姐：** 看来去 N 国还蛮危险的。

Miss Rivera: It seems Country N is a pretty dangerous place.

**医生：** 在旅行中，的确是有感染多种传染病的风险，但只要在旅行前做好充分的准备，进行必要的疫苗接种，携带一些预防药物，做好个人防护，是能够保证健康的。

Doctor: International travelers are often exposed to various infectious diseases, but you'll be fine as long as you prepare well and get necessary vaccination before the trip, bring some preventive medicines along, and have proper personal protection.

**Rivera 小姐：** 明白了。您刚才提到霍乱、疟疾、流行性脑膜炎等，都有什么预防方法吗？

Miss Rivera: I see. Do we have preventive measures against cholera, malaria, meningitis and other diseases that you've just mentioned?

**医生：** 有的。如避免昆虫、蚊虫叮咬，注意饮食卫生，备好必要的预防药物，注射流行性脑膜炎疫苗等。特别是疟疾在非洲很常见，而且目前疟疾没有疫苗可预防。疟疾是通过蚊虫叮咬传播的，所以防蚊措施不能马虎。

Doctor: Yes, we do. Prevent insect and mosquito bites, pay attention to food hygiene, prepare some preventive medicines, get the meningitis vaccine, and so on. Malaria, in particular, is widespread in Africa, but so far, no vaccine has been developed. Malaria is spread by the bite of an infected mosquito, so anti-mosquito measures are crucial.

**Rivera 小姐：** 可是蚊子这么小，终究防不胜防啊。

Miss Rivera: But mosquitoes are so tiny that it's impossible to keep them away at all times.

**医生：** 您不用太担心。只要您在确定旅游线路时避开疟疾的流行地区和流行季节，危险是可以降到最低的。另外，我还建议您携带适量的抗疟药品。

Doctor: Don't worry too much. As long as you avoid malaria-endemic areas and the transmission season when planning your travel itinerary, the risk of getting infected can be minimized. In addition, I suggest you take an appropriate amount of anti- malarial medicines with you.

**Rivera 小姐：** 抗疟药？这里有提供吗？

Miss Rivera: Anti-malarial medicines? Are they available here?

**医生：** 有的。我们提供的抗疟药是作为紧急治疗的备用药，它们的目的是治疗而不是预防。服药前要详细阅读说明书。感染者仍需尽快寻求医疗救治。

Doctor: Yes. We provide anti-malarial medicines as a backup of emergency treatment , and they're intended to treat rather than prevent malaria. Read the instructions carefully before taking the medicines. Infected people still need to seek medical attention as soon as possible.

**Rivera 小姐：** 明白了，您可真是给我上了一堂生动的课。我还以为去非洲就是看野生动物和大草原呢，没想到还有这么多要注意的。非常感谢您。

Miss Rivera: I see. Thank for very much for all the information. I thought that a visit to Africa was all about watching wild animals and exploring the grasslands, and I didn't expect that there is so much to learn. Thank you so much.

**医生：** 不客气。这是我们应该做的。再见。

Doctor: You're welcome. We're glad to have been of help. Goodbye.

**Rivera 小姐：** 再见！

Miss Rivera: Goodbye!

## 场景二　疫苗接种

SCENE 2: VACCINATION

---

**Elion 女士：** 您好，护士小姐，刚刚前台的医生建议我接种疫苗，是在这里吧？

Ms. Elion: Hello , nurse, the doctor at the front desk suggests that I get vaccinations, is this the right place?

**接种护士：** 是的，麻烦把您的申请单给我。我需要核对一下。

Vaccination Nurse: Yes, please give me your application form. I need to take a look first.

**Elion 女士：** 好的，给您。

Ms. Elion: Sure, here you are.

**接种护士：** 您是 Elion 女士，想接种黄热病、霍乱和流行性脑膜炎的疫苗，是吗？

Vaccination Nurse: You're Ms. Elion and you want to get vaccinations against yellow fever, cholera and epidemic meningitis, right?

**Elion 女士：** 是的。我是法国人，和我爱人在厦门工作。一个月后我计划去 N 国旅行，前台的医生说 N 国是一些重要传染病的流行区，建议我接种那三种疫苗以防感染。

Ms. Elion: Yes. I'm French and work here in Xiamen with my husband. I'm going to travel to Country N in a month, and the doctor at the front desk has just told me that some major infectious diseases are endemic in Country N, and he suggests I get those three vaccinations as a precaution.

**接种护士：** 是的，N 国在非洲西部，属热带草原气候，黄热病、流行性脑膜炎、霍乱等传染病时有流行，所以前台的杨医生建议您接种黄热病、霍乱和流行性脑膜炎疫苗。

Vaccination Nurse: Yes, Country N is in west Africa and has a savannah climate where infectious diseases such as yellow fever, cholera and epidemic meningitis are widespread, so Dr. Yang at the front desk suggests that you get vaccinations against yellow fever, cholera and epidemic meningitis.

**Elion 女士：** 明白了。那我现在可以接种了吗？

Ms. Elion: I see. So , can I get the vaccinations now?

**接种护士：** 我要先了解一下您是否有接种禁忌症。请问您现在身体是否不适？比如有没有感冒发热？

Vaccination Nurse: I need to know if you have any contraindications to vaccinations. Do you feel unwell at the moment? For example, do you have a cold or fever?

**Elion 女士：** 不瞒您说，我前几天感冒了，但现在已经好了。

Ms. Elion: To be honest , I caught a cold a few days ago, but I've recovered now.

**接种护士：** 好的，那您有无过敏史呢？

Vaccination Nurse: Okay, do you have any history of allergies?

**Elion 女士：** 没有过敏史。

Ms. Elion: No , I don't.

**接种护士：** 现在是否怀孕？或近期是否计划怀孕？

Vaccination Nurse: Are you pregnant now? Or do you plan to get pregnant in the near future?

**Elion 女士：** 没有怀孕，近期也没有计划怀孕。

Ms. Elion: I'm not pregnant and I have no plan to get pregnant in the near future.

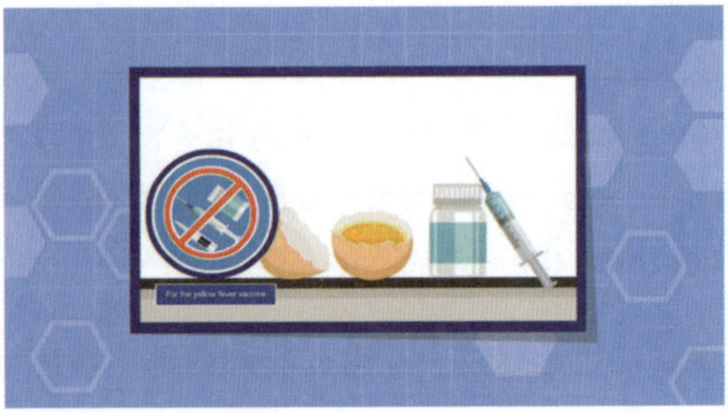

**接种护士：** 近一个月内有无接种过其他疫苗或者注射过免疫球蛋白？

Vaccination Nurse: Have you had any other vaccinations or immunoglobulin injections within the last month?

**Elion 女士：** 没有。

Ms. Elion: Nope.

**接种护士：** 好的，那我们开始接种了。请您脱去外衣，把左侧上臂露出来。我先为您接种黄热病疫苗，要从三角肌下缘进针。

Vaccination Nurse: Okay, let's start the vaccination. Please take off your coat and expose your left upper arm. I'll vaccinate you against yellow fever first; it'll be administered through the lower edge of the deltoid muscle.

**Elion 女士：** 说实话，我最怕打针。我已经十几年都没过打针了，您可千万轻一点啊！

Ms. Elion: Honestly, I have a fear of needles. I haven't had a shot in over 10 years, so please be gentle!

**接种护士：** 放心吧。也就一秒钟的事儿……好了，您按住棉球一两分钟，不出血后就可以把棉球扔到那边的黄色垃圾桶里。

Vaccination Nurse: Don't worry. It won't take a second... That's it; you can hold down the cotton ball for a minute or two, and then throw it into the yellow trash can over there after the bleeding stops.

**Elion 女士：** 已经打好了？真是没什么感觉。您还真是位高手呢！

Ms. Elion: That's it? I didn't feel anything. You're really good at this!

**接种护士：** 谢谢您的夸奖。现在为您接种流行性脑膜炎疫苗。

Vaccination Nurse: Thank you for your compliment. Now I'm going to give you the epidemic meningitis vaccine.

**Elion 女士：** 几种疫苗一起接种没有关系吗？

Ms. Elion: Is it okay for me to get multiple vaccine at the same time?

**接种护士：** 没有关系，在不同部位接种就可以了。请转身，把右侧上臂露出来……对，就是这样。

Vaccination Nurse: Don't worry, everything is fine as long as the injections are in different parts of the body. Please turn around and expose your right upper arm... Yes, that's right.

**Elion 女士：** 那还有一个疫苗怎么办？打哪里好呢？

Ms. Elion: What about the other vaccine? Where should it be injected?

**接种护士：** 还有一个是霍乱疫苗。它是口服胶囊，需要现场服用。您是第一次接种霍乱疫苗吗？

Vaccination Nurse: There is one more vaccine—the cholera vaccine. It is made up of oral capsules that must be taken on the spot. Is this your first cholera vaccination?

**Elion 女士：** 是的，第一次。

Ms. Elion: Yes, it is.

**接种护士：** 霍乱疫苗第一次接种须服 3 次，分别于 0 天、7 天、28 天口服，每次 1 粒。今天第 1 次服用。这是 1 粒霍乱疫苗，您现在就可以服用了，您右手边有饮水机和一次性水杯。

Vaccination Nurse: Cholera vaccine is given orally in three doses, each in a capsule, to be taken days 0, 7 and 28, respectively. Today, you're going to take the first dose. This is a cholera vaccine capsule and you can take it now. There is a water fountain and disposable cups to your right.

**Elion 女士：**（现场服用霍乱疫苗）这可方便多了。这就好了吗？

Ms. Elion: (Taking cholera vaccine on the spot) This is much more convenient. That's it?

**接种护士：** 从明天算起的第 7 天及第 28 天还需再各服 1 粒，这样您旅行前刚好都能服用完。

Vaccination Nurse: You need to take the second capsule on the 7th day counting from tomorrow and the third one on the 28th day; this means that you'll take them all before your trip.

**Elion 女士：**那我能带回去自己服用吗？

Ms. Elion: Can I bring them home and take them by myself?

**接种护士：**这疫苗需冷藏，一般情况下我们需要您到现场来。

Vaccination Nurse: The vaccine must be kept refrigerated and we usually need you to come here.

**Elion 女士：**哦……虽然是口服，还挺麻烦的啊。

Ms. Elion: Oh... though it's taken orally, it's quite troublesome.

**接种护士：**这样疫苗能规范保存，保护效果也更好。

Vaccination Nurse: This way the vaccine can be preserved and work better.

**Elion 女士：**明白了。那我现在可以走了吗？

Ms. Elion: I see. Can I leave now?

**接种护士：**您现在还不能离开。您需要在观察区观察半个小时。

Vaccination Nurse: We're not done yet. We need to keep you under observation for half an hour.

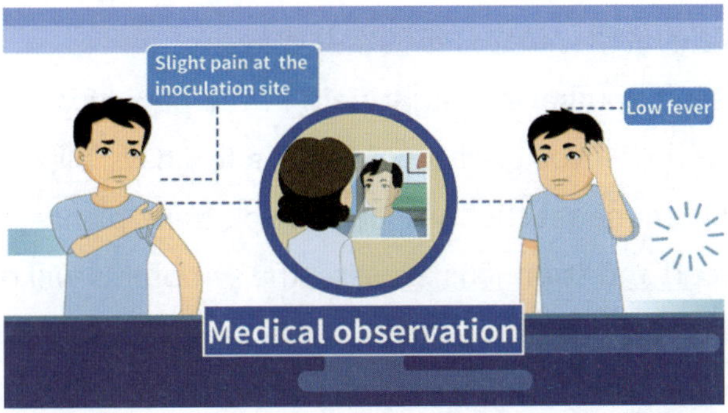


**Elion 女士：**这个应该没关系吧？我还想可以早点回单位呢。

Ms. Elion: It is really necessary to do so? I just want to get back to work as quickly as possible.

**接种护士：**这可不行。接种疫苗总的来说是安全的，但有一些人会出现头痛、肌肉痛、发热等不良反应，甚至出现严重的过敏反应需要急救。

Vaccination Nurse: Yes, it is. Vaccination is generally safe, but some people will have adverse reactions such as headache, muscle pain, fever, and even severe allergic reactions that require immediate medical attention.

**Elion 女士：** 哦，那还是听您的。

Ms. Elion: Okay, you're the expert.

**（半小时后）**

(Half an hour later)

**接种护士：** 接种后身体有没有不舒服？

Vaccination Nurse: Do you feel any discomfort after the vaccination?

**Elion 女士：** 没有。那接下来还有什么要注意的吗？

Ms. Elion: No , I don't. Is there anything else I should watch out for?

**接种护士：** 如果这几天出现接种部位轻微疼痛，或者低烧，不要紧张，属于正常的免疫反应。只要多喝水多休息，避免吃刺激性的食物，避免剧烈运动，一般三四天症状就会缓解或者消失。如果症状加重请立即拨打我们的咨询电话。这是疫苗接种注意事项的说明。请您仔细阅读并收好。

Vaccination Nurse: If you have a slight pain in the part of your body where the vaccine was injected, or if you get a low fever in a few days, please do not worry, as it's just a normal immune reaction. As long as you drink plenty of water, rest well and avoid spicy food and strenuous exercise, the symptoms will generally ease off or disappear in about three or four days. If the symptoms persist, please call our inquiry hotline immediately. This is a list of precautions for vaccination. Please read it carefully and keep it in a safe place.

**Elion 女士：** 好的。谢谢！

Ms. Elion: Okay. Thank you very much!

**接种护士：** 现在您可以离开了。离开前请凭您的证件到前台右侧的签证室领取预防接种证书。

Vaccination Nurse: You may leave now. Before you leave, you can pick up your vaccination certificate in the certification room to the right of the front desk.

**Elion 女士：** 好的。再见。

Ms. Elion: All right. Goodbye.

## 场景三 证书的签发、转签

SCENE 3: ISSUANCE AND TRANSFER OF CERTIFICATES

**签证医生：** 您好，有什么能帮到您的呢？

Certification Doctor: Hello , what can I do for you?

**Jolie 女士：** 您好，我的孩子在中国出生。在这里他已经打了许多预防针，这是他的接种记录。现在我丈夫在中国的任期已满，下个月我们全家就要回美国定居。在我们回家前您看我的孩子还需要接种什么疫苗吗？

Ms. Jolie: Hello! My child was born in China. He's got many vaccine shots here, here is his vaccination record. Now my husband's tenure in China has expired, and my family plans to return to the U.S. next month. What vaccines do you think my child needs before we head home?

**签证医生：** 好的，请坐，我看一下接种记录。很好，您的孩子现在 6 岁，已经按中国的计划免疫程序完成了接种。我们可以将您孩子的接种记录转录成英文。如果您希望您的孩子现在就按美国的计划免疫方案接种疫苗，今天还可以接种两针。

Certification Doctor: Okay, please take a seat, let me check the vaccination record. Well, your child is now 6 years old and has been vaccinated according to China's immunization program. We can transcribe this vaccination record into English. If you want your child to continue his vaccination according to the U. S. immunization program, he can get two shots today.

**Jolie 女士：** 谢谢您。能出具英文的接种证明会更好。您说还可以接种两针，那么是哪两针呢？

Ms. Jolie: Thank you. A vaccination certificate in English would be great. You've just said that my kid can get two shots, but what are the vaccines specifically?

**签证医生：** 一个是麻疹－腮腺炎－风疹疫苗，一个是水痘疫苗。

Certification Doctor: Measles–mumps–rubella and chickenpox vaccines.

**Jolie 女士：** 好的，我的孩子今天也来了。他身体正常，刚好可以接种这两针疫苗。

Ms. Jolie: Okay, my kid is with me here today. He's healthy and ready to get these two vaccine shots.

**签证医生：** 好的。您先带着孩子去接种疫苗，然后再来找我签发证书。

Certification Doctor: Great. Please take your child to get the shots first , and then come back to me for the certificate.

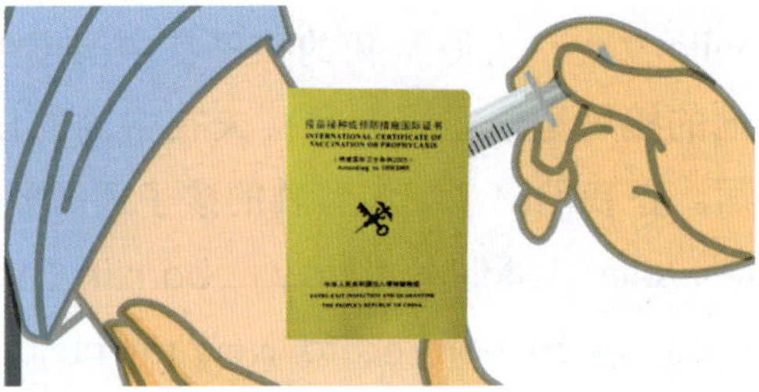

**Jolie 女士：** 谢谢，医生。

Ms. Jolie: Thank you very much, doctor.

**（接种完疫苗）**

(The child completes the vaccination)

**签证医生：** Jolie 女士，这是您孩子的疫苗接种或预防措施国际证书。刚才接种的疫苗都记录在里面了，中英文对照的，这就是"黄皮书"，已经盖章生效了。这是以前接种疫苗的转签记录。

Certification Doctor: Ms. Jolie, this is your child's "International Certificate of Vaccination or Prophylaxis". It includes the information on the vaccine shots he's just received, in both Chinese and English, and this is the "Yellow Book", stamped and effective. This is a transfer record of the previous vaccinations.

**Jolie 女士：** 太好了。谢谢你们。

Ms. Jolie: Wonderful. Thank you very much.

**签证医生：** 不客气。这是我们应该做的。

Certification Doctor: You're welcome. We're glad to have been of help.

# 第四节 旅行健康咨询
# SECTION V TRAVEL HEALTH CONSULTATION

## 场景一 旅行前健康评估
## SCENE 1: PRE-TRAVEL HEALTH ASSESSMENT

### 一、高血压旅行者旅行前健康评估
### 1. PRE- TRAVEL HEALTH ASSESSMENT FOR HYPERTENSIVE TRAVELERS

**医生：** 您好，有什么需要帮忙的吗？
Doctor: Hello , what can I do for you?

**Miller 先生：** 您好，我是在厦门工作的德国人，接下来我准备进行环球旅行。这是我的体检报告，想请医生帮我评估一下，我是否适合长途旅行。
Mr. Miller: Hello, I'm from Germany and I work here in Xiamen. I'm going to travel around the world. Here is my physical examination report. I'd like to have an assessment on whether I'm fit for long-distance travel.

**医生：** 好的。您做了一整套健康体检，很全面。体检结果显示您有轻度脂肪肝、高血压，还有肾结石。您目前有服用什么药物吗？
Doctor: Okay. You've completed a full set of physical examinations, with ever-ything covered. According to the report, you've got a low-grade fatty liver, hypert-ension and kidney stones. Are you taking any medications?

**Miller 先生：** 我一直在服用降压药。这样我可以出去旅游吗？
Mr. Miller: I've been taking anti-hypertensive drugs. Am I fit to travel?

**医生：** 从目前的检查结果来看，您可以出去旅游，但是旅行中要注意几点。首先是要严格按照医嘱服用降压药，确保血压维持在正常水平。
Doctor: Judging from the examination results, you can travel, and here're some tips for you. First of all, take anti-hypertensive drugs in strict accordance with the doctor's advice, and make sure your blood pressure stays at the normal level.

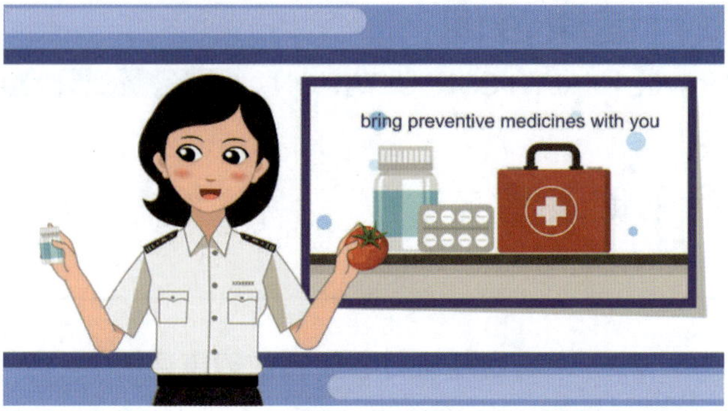


**Miller 先生：** 这个保证做到。我太太跟我一起出去，她会盯着我吃药的（笑）。

Mr. Miller: I'll do it. My wife's traveling with me, and she'll make sure that I take my medicines (laughing).

**医生：** 那很好。其次要保持心情舒畅，别给自己压力。

Doctor: That's great. And, be happy and don't stress yourself out.

**Miller 先生：** 那当然。出去旅游就是为了放松心情。

Mr. Miller: Absolutely. I'm traveling for pleasure.

**医生：** 飞机上空气比较干燥，长途飞行要注意补充液体；坐在座位上最好能活动下手脚，不要跷二郎腿，这样会妨碍血液循环。

Doctor: The air inside a plane cabin is very dry, you should drink plenty of water on long-haul flights; gently move your legs and arms from time to time while in the seat, and do not cross your legs as it'll hinder blood circulation.

**Miller 先生：** 嗯，很好的建议。有时候坐飞机时间长了，腿都会发麻。

Mr. Miller: Um, great advice. Some times my legs go numb during a long flight.

**医生：** 是的，一些情况下甚至会导致深静脉血栓呢。所以如果条件允许，最好每小时站起来并走动一会儿，可减少腿部血液淤滞和肿胀。

Doctor: Well, in some cases, even deep venous thrombosis can occur. So, if possible, stand up and move around for a while every hour to reduce blood stasis and swelling in the legs.

**Miller 先生：** 我会按您的建议做的。那有哪些病是不能进行长途旅行的呢？
Mr. Miller: I'll follow your advice. What medical conditions prevent people from traveling long distances?

**医生：** 患有一些疾病是不能长途旅行的，比如严重的心脏病、消化道出血、脑血管意外、癫痫病等。患有这些疾病的人，我们会建议他们取消长途旅行。
Doctor: People with certain medical conditions are not fit to travel long distances, such as severe heart diseases, gastrointestinal hemorrhage, cerebrovascular accident and epilepsy, etc. We suggest people with any of these medical conditions cancel their long-distance travel plans.

**Miller 先生：** 明白了。对了，医生，我过去几次国际旅行都有明显的时差反应，而且持续了好几天。您有没有什么建议呢？
Mr. Miller: I see. By the way, doctor, I had bad jetlag on my past few international trips, and it lasted a couple of days. Do you have any suggestions?

**医生：** 国际旅行时出现时差反应很正常，主要是要做好自我调整适应。
Doctor: Jetlag is a common problem for international travelers, and proper self-adjustment is very important.

**Miller 先生：** 这种感觉很不舒服，有时影响我的行程安排。我要怎么适应呢？
Mr. Miller: Some times, it gets so bad that it disrupts my travel itinerary. How can I adjust to it?

**医生：** 出发前和中长途旅行中要尽可能好好休息，即使是小睡一会儿对您也会很有帮助。到达后第一天一般会比较疲惫，建议不要做重大决定或开启紧张的旅行。
Doctor: Have a good rest before and during long-distance travels, and even a nap can be very helpful. On the first day after arrival, you'll usually feel tired, and it's definitely not the right time to make any big decision or start a stressful trip.

**Miller 先生：** 我在第一个晚上根本睡不着。怎么办呢？
Mr. Miller: I can't sleep at all on the first night. What should I do?

**医生：** 如果第一个晚上不能入睡，可以吃些钙片或一些含糖类的食品，如果汁或软糖，这样有助于睡意的产生。到达新的时区后，可以在清晨的阳光下散散步，以便刺激视神经，这有助于调节松果体中的生物钟。另外，还应试着按新的用餐时间进食。下午四点后建议少喝或不喝咖啡、茶或可乐。

Doctor: If you're sleepless on the first night, you can take some calcium tablets or eat sugary food, such as juice or chew candies, to help you fall asleep. After arriving in a new time zone, you can take a walk in the early morning sun to stimulate your optic nerves, as this will help regulate the body clock in the pineal gland. Also, try to adapt to the new meal times. Drink less or no coffee, tea or cola after 4 pm.

**Miller 先生：** 我知道了。经您这么介绍，我放心多了。多谢您！

Mr. Miller: I see. These tips put me at ease. Thank you very much.

**医生：** 不客气。

Doctor: You're welcome.

## 二、孕妇旅行前健康评估

## 2. PRE- TRAVEL HEALTH ASSESSMENT FOR PREGNANT WOMEN

**医生：** 您好，Aniston 小姐。

Doctor: Hello , Miss Aniston.

**Aniston 小姐：** 医生，我来自美国洛杉矶，在中国旅行了一个月。但是现在我发现我怀孕了，还能继续旅行吗？

Miss Aniston: Doctor, I'm from Los Angeles, USA, and I've been traveling around China for a month. But I've found that I'm pregnant. Can I continue traveling?

**医生：** 您怀孕几个月了？

Doctor: How long have you been pregnant?

**Aniston 小姐：** 2 个多月。

Miss Aniston: Over two months.

**医生：** 身体有没有不舒服？

Doctor: Do you feel any discomfort?

**Aniston 小姐**：没有，一切正常。

Miss Aniston: No , I feel perfectly well.

**医生**：一般情况下，在怀孕早期和晚期，建议避免旅行。

Doctor: Traveling during early or late pregnancy should be avoided if possible.

**Aniston 小姐**：那我是不是要等到 3 个月后才能旅行。

Miss Aniston: That means I should not travel until three months later.

**医生**：最好是这样。在怀孕中期，三个月到七个月这段时间，胎儿发育正常且较为稳定，是可以旅行的，但要密切注意身体变化，防止发生危险。同时在旅行时，应选择短途、安逸舒服的观光景点。在游玩过程中，应多注意休息，不要过于劳累，避免一些较剧烈的游乐项目。

Doctor: That's right. During mid-pregnancy, that is when you're three to seven months pregnant, you can travel if the fetus matures well, but you must watch out for any change in your body to prevent risks. Moreover, choose comfortable attractions which are not too far away. During your tours, take a break from time to time rather than tiring yourself out, and avoid vigorous recreational activities.

**Aniston 小姐**：我准备游览多个城市，需要多次乘坐飞机。乘飞机对孕妇有影响吗？

Miss Aniston: I'm going to visit several cities and need to take many flights. Is it safe to fly during pregnancy?

**医生**：以您目前的情况可以乘飞机旅行。但在飞行时每隔 1 ~ 2 小时要起来走动走动，多吃些蔬菜水果。

Doctor: Given your current situation, you're fit to travel by air. But you have to stand up and move around every one to two hours and eat more vegetables and fruits during the flight.

**Aniston 小姐**：我明白了，谢谢医生。

Miss Aniston: I see. Thank you very much, doctor.

**医生：**不客气。

Doctor: You're welcome.

## 场景二 旅行中健康状况的评估

SCENE 2: ASSESSMENT OF HEALTH STATUS DURING TRAVEL

**医生：**您好，这是国际旅行卫生保健中心，您有什么需要帮助的？

Doctor: Hello, this is the International Travel Healthcare Center, what can I do for you?

**Jackson 先生：**您好，我来自意大利，刚来中国留学不久。暑假的时候我准备在中国旅游一段时间。我想咨询一些旅行中需要注意的健康事项。

Mr. Jackson: Hello, I'm from Italy. I'm a new international student in China. I have plans to travel around the country during my summer break. I'd like to have some health advice for travelers.

**医生：**您计划去哪些地方旅行呢？

Doctor: Which places do you plan to visit?

**Jackson 先生：**我打算去内蒙古和西藏。这两个地方风光壮丽，不同于意大利。我已经向往很久了。

Mr. Jackson: I want to visit Inner Mongolia and Tibet. They have magnificent landscapes and are different Italy. I've been yearning to visit these two places for a long time.

**医生：**这两个地方可都是夏季的旅游热点，不过风土人情各有特色，旅游中需要注意的事项也有一些差别。您到内蒙古都去哪些地方呢？

Doctor: Both of them are very popular tourist destinations in summer, but they have different customs, and the tips for visits these two places are also different. Which places in Inner Mongolia are you going to visit?

**Jackson 先生：** 哦，我打算先去内蒙古呼伦贝尔大草原，在草原骑骑马。听说那里的马奶酒和手抓肉都很有民族特色，我也打算尝尝。

Mr. Jackson: Oh, I plan to go to the Hulunbeir Grassland first, where I'll try horse riding. I've heard that the local Kumis and boiled lamb are special ethnic foods, so I'd like to taste these delicacies.

**医生：** 总的来说，内蒙古属于半干旱半湿润的温带季风气候，夏季是去内蒙古旅游的最佳季节。您的计划很棒。

Doctor: In general, Inner Mongolia has a semi-arid and semi-humid temperate monsoon climate, and summer is the best time to tour Inner Mongolia. You've got great plans.

**Jackson 先生：** 是啊，我也很期待。但我看路上的时间较长，我怕我会晕车。有没有什么办法呢？

Mr. Jackson: Right, I'm looking forward to the trip, but I'm afraid that I may get motion sickness since I'll have to spend much time on the road. Do you have good advice?

**医生：** 内蒙古旅游景点比较分散，旅游线路长。尽量坐在车的前座。路上可以听听音乐，必要时可以准备一些晕车药品。另外，在旅游途中还要注意补充水分，内蒙古草原饮水含碱量高，记得不要喝生水。

Doctor: In Inner Mongolia, the major sights and attractions are spread out across the region, and the tour routes are pretty long. Try to get a front seat on the bus. Listen to some music while on the road, and if necessary, bring some anti-motion sickness medicines with you. Besides, drink plenty of water during travel. Water on Inner Mongolia's grasslands has a high level of alkalinity, so don't drink water straight from the tap.

**Jackson 先生：** 好的，我想到时租个车，多带点瓶装水就好了。

Mr. Jackson: Okay, I'll rent a car and bring plenty of bottled water.

**医生：** 此外我看您的几个目的地都在牧区，还需要注意防范“旅行者腹泻”和一些人畜共患病。

Doctor: Besides, I've noticed that several of your destinations are in pastoral areas. You need t o guard against "traveler's diarrhea" and some zoonosis.

**Jackson 先生：** 您说的这都是什么病啊。怎么好像没听过？

Mr. Jackson: I've no idea what they mean. I don't think I've ever heard of them?

**医生：** "旅行者腹泻"是旅行中最常见的病症之一，俗称"水土不服"。通常表现为每天拉肚子 3 次或 3 次以上，或者同时有发热、腹痛或呕吐等症状。

Doctor: "Traveler's diarrhea", commonly known as "non-acclimatization", is one of the most common illnesses among travelers. The sufferer often has three or more bowel movements a day, or develop symptoms such as fever, abdominal pain or vomiting.

**Jackson 先生：** 哦，原来是拉肚子啊……上次我去印度旅游一路上拉了好几天肚子，严重影响了我的旅游安排。那是再糟糕不过的经历了，我可不想再碰到。

Mr. Jackson: Oh, so it's diarrhea... I had diarrhea for a couple of days during my visit to India, and my tour plan was seriously disrupted. That was my worst experience ever, and I definitely don't want to have it again.

**医生：** 是啊。在过去，人们认为"旅行者腹泻"是因为对当地的气候、食物等不习惯引起的。事实上，它一般是由细菌、病毒、肠道寄生虫等致病微生物导致的急性肠道传染病。

Doctor: You're right. In the past, "traveler's diarrhea" was thought to be caused by inability to adapt to local climate and food. In fact, it's usually an acute intestinal infectious disease caused by pathogenic microorganisms, such as b acteria, viruses and intestinal parasites.

**Jackson 先生：** 哦，还会传染啊。那要怎么预防呢？

Mr. Jackson: Oh, it's infectious. How can we protect ourselves against it?

**医生：** 首先要保持良好的个人卫生习惯，确保饮食、饮水卫生。刚才说了不喝生水，也尽量不要吃生冷食物；水果吃前要清洗、去皮；餐前便后及接触脏东西后要洗手；气候变化时注意增减衣物，诸如此类的。您还可以酌情带些口服补液盐或抗生素以备不时之需。

Doctor: First of all, keeping good personal hygiene and avoid unhygienic foodstuffs and drinks. As I said just now, don't drink water straight from the tap, and avoid raw or cold food; wash and peel fruits before eating them; wash your hands before meals, after going to the bathroom, or after touching dirty things; dress right for the weather, and so on. You may also bring some oral rehydration salts or antibiotics, just in case.

**Jackson 先生：** 明白了。那您刚才提到的另外一种病是什么呢？听起来好像跟动物有关。

Mr. Jackson: I see. What is the other disease you mentioned just now? It sounds like it has some thing to do with animals.

**医生：** 哈哈，您很聪明，确实是这样。人畜共患病是人类和脊椎动物之间自然感染与传播的疾病，比如狂犬病、炭疽病和一些寄生虫病。

Doctor: Ha-ha, you're very smart, that's right. Zoonoses are defined as those diseases and infections which are naturally transmitted between vertebrate animals and humans, such as rabies, anthracnose and certain parasitic diseases.

**Jackson 先生：** 听起来很可怕的。它们能从动物传染给人类吗？

Mr. Jackson: Sounds horrible. Are they transmissible from animals to humans?

**医生：** 简单来说是这样没错。被患病的动物咬伤，接触它们的排泄物、皮毛，以及加工病畜肉或食用未煮熟的畜肉等途径都有可能感染。

Doctor: Absolutely true. A person is likely to catch this disease if he gets bitten by an infected animal or is exposed to its feces or fur, handles its meat, or eat under cooked animal meat.

**Jackson 先生：** 那我还能不能骑马啊？

Mr. Jackson: Then can I still try horse riding?

**医生：** 您也不用太担心。关键是要做好必要的防护措施。除了良好的个人卫生习惯之外，在牧区还要注意尽量不要饮用生乳，不吃未煮熟的畜肉，避免与动物近距离接触……

Doctor: Don't worry. The point is to take necessary precautions. Besides keeping good personal hygiene, avoid drinking raw milk, eating undercooked meat, and coming into close contact with animals in pastoral areas...

**Jackson 先生：**啊……我还准备跟大草原上的牛羊群们亲密接触一下呢，最好还能邂逅很萌的土拨鼠。

Mr. Jackson: Ah... I thought I could get close to the cattle and sheep on the grasslands and even meet the cute marmots.

**医生：**任意与动物拥抱、亲吻等，是有可能从它们身上染上人畜共患病。身上皮肤有破损时更要倍加小心。特别要防止被动物咬伤、抓伤。有些动物可不像您想象的那么温和。

Doctor: Hugging or kissing animals carelessly may expose you to zoonoses. Be especially careful if you have cracked skin. In particular, avoid getting bitten and scratched by an animal. Some animals aren't as gentle as you might think.

**Jackson 先生：**好吧，我记下了。那去西藏要注意些什么呢？

Mr. Jackson: Well, I'll keep that in mind. Are there any tips for traveling to Tibet?

**医生：**西藏的旅游线路很长，牧区也多，所以刚才提到的很多注意事项在西藏也是适用的。另外，西藏地处青藏高原，平均海拔在 4000 米以上，空气比较稀薄，日晒较强烈。因此还要注意防范高山病以及晒伤。

Doctor: Tibet has long tour routes and many pastoral areas too, so many of the precautions just mentioned are also useful in Tibet. Besides, Tibet is located on the Qinghai-Tibet Plateau, rising more 4,000 meters above sea level. The air is thin, and the sun is strong. So, you need to protect yourself from high-altitude illness and sunburn.

**Jackson 先生：**嗯，在意大利，我有一些朋友经常徒步攀登阿尔卑斯山脉，听他们说起有些人会有高原反应，出现一些症状。有报道称，一些严重的甚至丢了性命。说实话，我心里有点忐忑不安，毕竟我之前没有到过高海拔地区。

Mr. Jackson: Well, in Italy, I have some friends who often go hiking in the Alps, and they've told me that some people are vulnerable to altitude sickness and show some symptoms. There are reports of fatality in some serious cases. To be honest, I'm a little worried because I've never been to high-altitude areas before.

**医生：**是的。有些人到了高海拔地区会出现恶心、头痛、睡眠障碍、厌食、全身倦怠、呼吸困难等症状。严重的甚至出现高原肺水肿、脑水肿等危及生命的紧急状况。

Doctor: It's true. Some people experience symptoms like nausea, headache, sleep disorders, anorexia, general malaise and shortness of breath when they're in a high-altitude area. In serious cases, they may even face life-threatening conditions, such as high-altitude pulmonary edema and cerebral edema.

**Jackson 先生：**那怎么办？我还能去西藏吗？

Mr. Jackson: What shall I do? Can I still visit Tibet?

**医生：**您也不用太担心。其实几乎所有的严重高原病都是可以预防的。关键是要对它有充分了解，并采取措施。防患于未然。

Doctor: Don't worry too much. In fact, almost all severe altitude-illnesses are preventable. It's crucial to gain a full understanding of them and take the relevant measures. Prevention is better than cure.

**Jackson 先生：**我迫不及待地想听您给我仔细讲讲。

Mr. Jackson: I can't wait to hear more about it.

**医生：**避免高原反应要有一个适应过程。阶梯式上山是预防急性高原病最稳妥、最安全的方法。像您这样的初入高山者一般应在海拔 2500～3000 米的地方停留两三天，然后每天上升的速度不宜超过 600～900 米。

Doctor: It takes time to adapt to high altitudes and prevent altitude-illness. Going up the mountain step by step is the most proper and safest way to prevent acute altitude illness. A beginner like you should usually stay at an altitude of 2500 to

3000 meters for two or three days, and then go up by no more than 600 to 900 meters every day afterwards.

**Jackson 先生：** 2500～3000 米？那什么地方合适呢？

Mr. Jackson: 2500 to 3000 meters? Which place would that be?

**医生：** 我认为林芝是个不错的选择，您可以参考一下。

Doctor: I think Nyingchi is a good choice, and you may consider it.

**Jackson 先生：** 我的中国同学向我推荐过这地方，听说很美丽。我再做做旅游攻略，仔细规划一下路线。

Mr. Jackson: My Chinese classmates have recommended this place to me, and I've heard that it is a beautiful place. I'll do more research and plan my travel itinerary.

**医生：** 到达高原的第一个 24 小时，要避免过度劳累和饮酒，并应增加饮水量。

Doctor: In the first 24 hours after arriving at the highland, avoid tiring yourself out and drinking wine, and take plenty of water.

**Jackson 先生：** 哦，我本来还打算和同行的朋友到了之后小酌两杯庆祝一下呢。看来不行了。

Mr. Jackson: Oh, I've planned to have some drinks with my friends to celebrate the trip after arrival. It seems this isn't a good idea.

**医生：** 是啊，要等适应当地海拔高度之后再考虑。如果出现剧烈的高原反应，千万不能继续去更高海拔的地方。应停留在原海拔位置，直到症状消失。

Doctor: Yeah. Don't think about it until you have got used to the altitude. If you suffer from severe altitude sickness, don't venture into higher-altitude areas. Stay where you are until your symptoms have disappeared.

**Jackson 先生：** 如果没有消失怎么办呢？

Mr. Jackson: What if the symptoms persist?

**医生：** 如果高原反应的症状严重或持续时间超过 2 天，或者有进行性呼吸困难伴有咳嗽、疲劳，甚至出现走路不稳不协调等病情恶化情况，应及时就医。

Doctor: You should see the doctor immediately, if the symptoms of altitude sickness are serious or last over two days, or if you feel progressive shortness of breath with cough, fatigue or even signs of worsening conditions, such as staggering or abalance disorder.

**Jackson 先生：**看来不能掉以轻心啊……那有什么可以急用的药物吗？
Mr. Jackson: It seems that we can't take it lightly... Is there any medicine that we can take in an emergency?

**医生：**可以携带一些抗高原反应的药物，如乙酰唑胺、阿司匹林、地塞米松等，以备不时之需。
Doctor: You can bring some anti-altitude sickness medicines, such as acetazolamide, aspirin and dexamethasone, just in case.

**Jackson 先生：**明白了。听说拉萨被称为“阳光城”，那里阳光一定很充沛吧？
Mr. Jackson: I see. I've heard that Lhasa is known as the "City of Sunlight", there must be plenty of sunshine there, right?

**医生：**是的，阳光无限好，但是晒多了也不行。要注意防止晒伤和视力损伤。
Doctor: Yes, it is. There is beautiful sunlight, but too much sun exposure can have serious consequences. Avoid sunburns and protect your eyes in the sun.

**Jackson 先生：**这个我有经验。在意大利的时候我也经常去海边晒太阳。
Mr. Jackson: I have experience with this. When I was in Italy, I often headed to the beach for sunbathing.

**医生：**高海拔地区空气稀薄，紫外线更强。特别是有计划到雪山去旅游探险的，更不能掉以轻心。
Doctor: In high-altitude areas, the air is thin and the ultraviolet rays are strong. You should be very cautious if you plan to explore the snowy mountains.

**Jackson 先生：**必须戴墨镜和抹防晒霜，对吧？
Mr. Jackson: I have to put on sunglasses and sunscreens, right?

**医生：** 这是两种有效的防护措施，但最好穿着能遮蔽手背和腿部的衣物，这比涂防晒霜的效果要好得多。另外，在紫外线最强烈的中午时段最好不要外出，在水上和雪地里要采取措施避免过度暴晒。

Doctor: These are two effective protective measures, but make sure that your clothing covers your hands and legs, which is more effective than sunscreens. In addition, it's best not to go out at noon when the ultraviolet rays are strongest, and take measures against excessive sun exposure on the water and snow lands.

**Jackson 先生：** 那墨镜和防晒霜有什么特殊要求吗？

Mr. Jackson: Are there any special requirements for sunglasses and sunscreens?

**医生：** 您可以选择包围式的紫外线防护墨镜，并配以宽边太阳帽。防晒霜最好选择防晒因子（SPF）大于 15 的，对没有衣物保护的暴露部位，要经常重复涂抹。

Doctor: You can wear UV protection wrap-around sunglasses and a broad-brimmed sunhat. A sunscreen with an SPF greater than 15 is preferred, and you should reapply sunscreen on exposed skin from time to time.

**Jackson 先生：** 没想到旅行中这么多问题需要注意。这次咨询对我真是受益匪浅，太谢谢您了。

Mr. Jackson: I didn't expect that there are so many tips for traveling. All the information is very useful. Thank you so much.

**医生：** 不客气。也预祝您旅途愉快，身体健康。

Doctor: You're welcome. I wish you a pleasant journey and good health.

## 场景三 旅行后健康状况的评估

SCENE 3: POST-TRAVEL HEALTH ASSESSMENT

**医生：** 您好，有什么需要帮助的吗？

Doctor: Hello , do you need any help?

**Miller 先生：** 您好，我是在厦门工作的德国人。我刚从东南亚旅行回来，旅行前我记得这里的医生建议我旅行回来要进行健康评估。您可以帮我吗？
Mr. Miller: Hello, I'm a German working here in Xiamen. I've just returned from a trip to Southeast Asia. I remember that, before the trip, a doctor here suggested that I have a health assessment when I come back. Can you help me with that?

**医生：** 当然可以。东南亚是旅游的好地方。您都去了哪些地方？旅行了多长时间？
Doctor: Sure. Southeast Asia is a great place for sightseeing. Which cities did you visit , and how long was your trip?

**Miller 先生：** 我先去了泰国的芭堤雅，接着去了越南的胡志明，还去了马来西亚吉隆坡，最后去了印度尼西亚的巴厘岛。整个行程 15 天。
Mr. Miller: I headed to Pattaya in Thailand first and then I visited Ho Chi Minh City in Vietnam, Kuala Lumpur in Malaysia, and finally Bali in Indonesia. The entire trip took 15 days.

**医生：** 很不错的行程！在旅行中有没有出现身体不适的情况？
Doctor: What a great trip! Did you feel unwell during the trip?

**Miller 先生：** 在 V 国的时候拉了几天肚子，后来就好了。不过那边的蚊子很多，大部分是那种身上有白点的花蚊子。咬起人可凶了，我是被咬了好几次。
Mr. Miller: I had diarrhea for a couple of days in Country V, but I recovered shortly afterwards. There were just too many mosquitoes, and most of them were "A sian tiger mosquitoes" with white spots on their bodies. They were ferocious biters, and I got bitten quite a few times.

**医生：** 旅行中有没有服用过什么药物呢？
Doctor: Did you take any medicines during the trip?

**Miller 先生：** 拉肚子的时候吃了两天抗生素，好了之后就没再继续吃了。
Mr. Miller: I took antibiotics for two days when I had diarrhea, and I stopped taking them after I recovered.

**医生：** 旅行过程中出现腹泻症状是最常见的旅行健康问题之一，必要的时候服用抗生素是对的。那被蚊子咬了以后，有没有出现异常的症状？

Doctor: Diarrhea is one of the most common illnesses among travelers, and taking antibiotics when necessary is the right thing to do. Did you have any unusual symptoms after being bitten by mosquitoes?

**Miller 先生：**这也是我来找医生的原因。我旅行回来后，感觉很疲劳，全身酸痛。昨晚出现 37.3℃的低热，今天早上有点头痛、恶心和眼眶痛。

Mr. Miller: That's why I'm here today. Since I came back from the trip, I've been feeling very tired and sore all over. Last night, I had a low fever of 37.3℃, and this morning, I got a headache with nausea and orbital pain.

**医生：**身上有没有皮疹？或者出现牙龈出血、流鼻血等症状？

Doctor: Do you have a rash on your body? Or have you got symptoms such as gum bleeding and nosebleeds?

**Miller 先生：**在旅行中有身上有好几个地方很痒，但是也没什么其他特别的症状。这几天我太太说我脖子和胸前皮肤有点发红，不知道是不是过敏了。还有这两天刷牙的时候牙龈出血，我以为是牙刷的问题。

Mr. Miller: I didn't have unusual symptoms except that I felt itchy in several parts of my body during the trip. My wife said that my neck and chest flush slightly these days, and I'm not sure if it is allergy. Also, when I brush my teeth these two days, my gums bleed. I thought it was the toothbrush to blame.

**医生：**根据您的旅行史和症状，您有可能是感染了登革热。我们需要给您进行必要的检查，才能确诊。请跟我来。

Doctor: Judging from your travel history and symptoms, you may have dengue fever. We need to do more diagnostic tests. Please follow me.

**（抽血检查）**

(Blood test)

**医生：**您好，根据您的旅行史、临床症状和血样检测结果，我们可以确认您感染了登革热。

Doctor: Hello, based on your travel history, clinical symptoms and blood test results, we can confirm that you have dengue fever.

**Miller 先生：**登革热？是什么病？
Mr. Miller: Dengue fever? What is it?

**医生：**登革热是由登革热病毒引起的由蚊虫传播的急性传染病。患者常常会出现突发发热，全身肌肉、骨、关节痛，疲乏，皮疹等症状。
Doctor: Dengue fever is a mosquito-borne acute infectious disease caused by the dengue virus. Patients often have symptoms like a sudden fever,systemic muscle, bone, joint pain, fatigue and rash.

**Miller 先生：**就是说这个病是因为被蚊子叮咬而感染上的？
Mr. Miller: Do you mean that this disease is caused by mosquit obites?

**医生：**是的。这种病在东南亚国家呈地方性流行，您刚才提到的那种“花蚊子”很可能就是本病的传播媒介“白纹伊蚊”。如果被携带有病毒的蚊子叮咬，就可能被感染。
Doctor: Yes. This disease is endemic in Southeast Asia. The “A sian tiger mosquitoes” you just mentioned might be Aedes albopictus, the transmission vector of this disease. If you get bitten by a mosquito carrying the virus, you may be infected.

**Miller 先生：**那我会不会传给我家人啊？
Mr. Miller: Is it possible that I pass the disease on to my family?

**医生：**白纹伊蚊在中国南方也是常见蚊种之一，所以理论上也是有可能的。建议您让家人也注意自我健康监测。如有必要的话，到我们中心或者医院做个检测。
Doctor: Aedes albopictus is also a common mosquito species in South China, so it is theoretically possible. I suggest that your family keep a close eye on self-health condition. If necessary, you guys can come to our center or the hospital for examinations.

**Miller 先生：**好的。原来蚊子就是罪魁祸首……那这种病严重吗？
Mr. Miller: Okay. It turns out that mosquitoes are to blame... Is this disease serious?

**医生：** 登革热是一种具有自限性倾向的传染性疾病，通常预后良好。但少部分患者会出现出血热症状，甚至出现休克、多器官功能衰竭甚至死亡的情况。

Doctor: Dengue fever is a self-limited infectious disease with generally favorable prognosis. However, a small percentage of patients develop symptoms of hemorrhagic fever, and there are even reports of shock, multiple organ failure and even fatality.

**Miller 先生：** 这么严重。那我现在怎么办呢？

Mr. Miller: That's terrible. What should I do now?

**医生：** 目前没有特效药，只能对症治疗。鉴于您目前的病情，我建议您带着我们的检测报告尽快到正规医院进行对症治疗。不过不用太担心，您只要积极配合医生的治疗，很快就能痊愈。

Doctor: There is no specific medicine available, and symptomatic treatment is the only solution. Given your current condition, I suggest you take our test report to a reputable hospital for symptomatic treatment as soon as possible. But don't worry too much, as long as you follow the doctor's advice and undergo the treatment with a positive attitude, you'll recover soon.

**Miller 先生：** 看来今天真是来对了。经过您的检查和诊断，我也放心了。我现在就去 XX 医院治疗。

Mr. Miller: It's the right move for me to come here today. Your test and diagnosis have put me at ease. I'm heading to XX Hospital for treatment.

**医生：** 非常好，我给您开了张就诊方便卡。您拿着这张卡可以直接找医生看病。

Doctor: Very good, I'll give you a "Medical Convenience Card". With this card, you can go straight to the doctor.

**Miller 先生：** 太好了，谢谢医生。再见。

Mr. Miller: Great, thank you very much, doctor. Goodbye.

**医生：** 再见，祝您早日康复！

Doctor: Goodbye and I wish you a quick recovery!

# 附　录

APPENDIX

# （一）有关机构和团体

## （Ⅰ）Relevant Institufions and Groups

1. **世界卫生组织（世卫组织）**
   World Health Organization（WHO）
2. **世卫组织驻华代表处**
   WHO China Representative Office
3. **国际旅行者医疗救助协会**
   International Association for Medical Assistance to Travellers
4. **国家卫生健康委员会（国家卫生健康委）**
   National Health Commission (NHC)
5. **中国疾病预防控制中心（中国疾控中心）**
   Chinese Center for Disease Control and Prevention (China CDC)
6. **中国红十字会** Red Cross Society of China
7. **中国海关** China Customs
8. **国家移民管理局** National Immigration Administration
9. **公安部** Ministry of Public Security
10. **领事馆** Consulate
11. **航空公司** Airlines

# （二）有关人员名称

## （Ⅱ）Name of Relevant Personnel

12. **驾驶员 / 机械师 / 列车长 / 列车员**
    Driver/Mechanic/Train Conductor/Train Crew
13. **国际旅客** International Passenger
14. **国内旅客** Domestic Passenger
15. **转机旅客** Connecting Passenger

16. **过境旅客** Transit Passenger
17. **残疾旅客** Handicapped Passenger
18. **出港旅客** Departing Passenger
19. **进港旅客** Arriving Passenger
20. **代理** Agent
21. **主任** Chief
22. **经理** Manager
23. **机组人员** Flight Crew
24. **机长** Captain
25. **飞行员** Pilot
26. **正驾驶员** First Pilot
27. **副驾驶员** Copilot/Second Pilot
28. **女乘务员 / 男乘务员** Stewardess/Steward
29. **乘务长** Purser/Chief Attendant
30. **地勤人员** Ground Crew
31. **检疫员** Quarantine Doctor
32. **消毒员** Disinfection Worker
33. **检验员** Inspector/Surveyor
34. **安全员** Safety Officer
35. **船长** Captain/Master
36. **大副** Chief Officer / First Mate
37. **二副** Second Officer / Second Mate
38. **三副** Third Officer / Third Mate
39. **水手长** Bosun
40. **一水** Able-Bodied Sailor (AB)
41. **二水** Ordinary Sailor (OS)
42. **普通水手** Seaman
43. **木匠** Carpenter
44. **轮机长 / 老轨** Chief Engineer
45. **大管轮** Second Engineer

46. **二管轮** Third Engineer
47. **三管轮** Fourth Engineer
48. **电机员** Electrical Engineer
49. **加油工** Oiler
50. **钳工** Fitter
51. **大厨** Chief Cook
52. **餐厅服务员** Mess Boy
53. **确诊病例** Confirmed Cases
54. **疑似病例** Suspected Cases
55. **有症状人员** Symptomatic Person
56. **无症状携带者 / 感染者** Asymptomatic Carrier / Infected Person
57. **密切接触者** Close Contact
58. **宿主** Host
59. **易感人群** Susceptible/Vulnerable Population
60. **重症患者** Patients in Severe or Critical Condition
61. **轻症患者** Patients with Mild Symptoms

## （三）交通工具结构与设施

### （Ⅲ）Structure and Facilities of Transportation Vehicles

62. **前 / 中 / 后 / 尾舱** Fore/Mid/Back/Rear Cabin
63. **驾驶舱** Wheel House/ Cockpit
64. **客舱** Passenger Cabin
65. **货舱** Hold
66. **头等舱** First Class
67. **公务舱** Business Class
68. **经济舱** Economy/Tourist Class
69. **配膳间** Pantry

70. **登机门** Entry Door
71. **行李架** Luggage Rack
72. **更衣室** Locker Room
73. **卫生间** Toilet/Lavatory/Washroom/Restroom
74. **马桶** Water Closet
75. **机上广播系统** In-flight Announc ement System

## （四）口岸有关区域与设施

### ( IV ) Relevant Areas and Facilities of Ports

76. **半污染区 / 清洁区 / 污染区**
    Clean / Partially Contaminated / Contaminated Area
77. **红外测温区** Infrared Temperature Measurement Area
78. **流行病调查室** Epidemiological Investigation Room
79. **医学排查室** Medical Screening Room
80. **采样间** Sampling Room
81. **负压室** Negative Pressure Room
82. **患者专用通道** Entrance/Corridor for Patients
83. **入口 / 出口** Entrance/Exit
84. **自动门** Automatic Door
85. **自动扶梯 /（升降式）电梯** Escalator/Elevator
86. **自动步道** Moving /Automatic Walkway
87. **登机廊桥** Air Bridge
88. **9 号登机口** Boarding Gate No.9
89. **机场大厦 / 候机楼** Terminal Departure Building
90. **国内 / 国际** Domestic/International
91. **到达 / 离港** Arrivals/Departures
92. **大厅** Lobby/Lounge

**93. 航班显示板** Flight Information Board
**94. 失物招领处** Lost & Found
**95. 行李认领区** Baggage Claim Area
**96. 行李寄存** Left Luggage
**97. 母婴室** Nursery
**98. 免税商店** Duty-Free Shop
**99. 自动取款机** ATM
**100. 值机柜台** Check-In Counter
**101. 中转柜台** Transfer Counter
**102. 安检柜台** Security Counter
**103. 问询处** Information Counter / Inquiry Office
**104. 急救中心** First Aid Counter
**105. 定点医院** Designated Hospital

## （五）有关单证材料

## （V）Relevant Documents

**106. 总申报单 / 旅客舱单 / 货物舱单**
General Declaration / Passenger Manifest / Cargo Manifest
**107. 货物申报单** Cargo Declaration
**108. 压舱水清单** Ballast List
**109. 机组（船员）名单 / 旅客名单** Crew List / Passenger List
**110. 护照** Passport
**111. 行程单** Itinerary
**112. 中华人民共和国出 / 入境健康申明卡**
Exit/Entry Health Declaration Form of the People's Republic of China
**113. 健康申明卡** Health Declaration Form
**114. 流行病学调查表** Epidemiological Survey Form

**115. 采样知情同意书** Informed Consentfor Sampling

**116. 关封** Customs Cover

**117. 船舶免予卫生控制措施证书**

Ship Sanitation Control Exemption Certificate

**118. 船舶卫生控制措施证书**

Ship Sanitation Control Certificate

**119. 船舶入境检疫证** Pratique

**120. 入境卫生检疫证书** Free Pratique

**121. 检疫处理通知书**

Notification of Inspection and Quarantine Treatment

**122. 航海健康申报书** Maritime Declaration of Health

**123. 港序列表** Ports of Call List

**124. 船员名单** Crew List

**125. 旅客名单** Passenger List

**126. 疫苗接种名单** Vaccination List

**127. 船用物品申报单** Ship's Stores Declaration

**128. 航次备忘录** Voyage Memo

**129. 垃圾管理计划** Garbage Management Plan

**130. 压舱水管理计划** Ballast Water Management Plan

**131. 饮用水分析报告** Drinking Water Analysis Report

**132. 食品供应清单** Food Supply List

**133. 医疗记录本** Medical Logbook

**134. 药品合格证明** Certificate for Medicines

**135. 疫苗接种或预防措施国际证书**

International Certificate of Vaccination or Prophy Laxis

**136. 健康证书** Health Certificate

# （六）疾病名称

## （VI）Disease Name

137. 鼠疫 / 肺鼠疫 / 腺鼠疫 / 败血症鼠疫

Plague / Pneumonic Plague / Bubonic Plague / Septicemic Plague

138. 霍乱 Cholera

139. 黄热病 Yellow Fever

140. 新型冠状病毒感染 COVID-19

141. 严重急性呼吸综合征

Severe Acute Respiratory Syndrome (SARS)

142. 中东呼吸综合征

Middle East Respiratory Syndrome (MERS)

143. 人感染高致病性禽流感

Human Infection with Highly Pathogenic Avian Influenza

144. 甲型 H1N1 流感 Influenza A (H1N1)

145. 人感染 H7N9 禽流感

Human Infection with H7N9 Avian Influenza

146. 肺炭疽 Lung Anthrax

147. 肺结核 Pulmonary Tuberculosis

148. 流行性脑脊髓膜炎 Epidemic Cerebrospinal Meningitis

149. 细菌性痢疾 Bacillary Dysentery

150. 肠出血性大肠杆菌 O157:H7 感染性腹泻

Enterohemorrhagic Escherichia Coli O157:H7 Infectious Diarrhea

151. 诺如病毒感染 Norovirus Infection

152. 副溶血性弧菌感染 Paralytic Vibrio Infection

153. 登革热 Dengue Fever

154. 疟疾 Malaria

155. 流行性乙型脑炎 Japanese Encephalitis

156. 埃博拉出血热 Ebola Hemorrhagic Fever

157. 西尼罗热 West Nile fever
158. 基孔肯亚热 Chikungunya Fever
159. 寨卡病毒病 Zika Virus Disease
160. 裂谷热 Rift Valley Fever
161. 马尔堡出血热 Marburg Hemorrhagic Fever
162. 拉沙热 Lassa Fever
163. 天花 Smallpox
164. 梅毒 Syphilis
165. 性病 Venereal Disease
166. 水痘 Chicken Pox
167. 麻疹 Measles
168. 风疹 Rubella
169. 腮腺炎 Mumps
170. 白喉 Diphtheria
171. 百日咳 Pertussis
172. 破伤风 Tetanus
173. 伤寒 Typhoid
174. 肺炎 Pneumonia
175. 高血压 Hypertension/ High Blood Pressure
176. 糖尿病 Diabetes
177. 冠心病 Coronary Heart Disease
178. 动脉硬化 Arteriosclerosis
179. 哮喘 Asthma
180. 食物中毒 Food Poisoning
181. 中暑 Heat Stroke
182. 心脏病 Heart Disease
183. 心肌梗死 Myocardial Infarction
184. 过敏 Allergy
185. 睡眠障碍 Sleep Disorder

# （七）常见症状

## （Ⅶ）Common Symptoms

**186. 发热** Fever
**187. 寒战** Chills
**188. 乏力** Fatigue
**189. 咳嗽** Cough
**190. 干咳** Dry Cough
**191. 呼吸困难** Dyspnea / Breathing Difficulties
**192. 鼻塞** Stuffy Nose
**193. 流涕** Runny Nose
**194. 头痛** Headache
**195. 咽痛** Sore Throat
**196. 胸痛** Chest Pain
**197. 肌肉痛** Muscle/Joint Pain
**198. 关节痛** Arthralgia
**199. 恶心呕吐** Nausea and Vomiting
**200. 腹泻** Diarrhea
**201. 黄疸** Jaundice
**202. 腹痛** Abdominal Pain
**203. 皮疹** Rash
**204. 呼吸道症状** Respiratory Symptom
**205. 消化道症状** Gastrointestinal Symptom
**206. 蚊媒传染病症状** Mosquito-Borne Disease Symptom

## （八）常用药名

### （Ⅷ）Common Drugs

207. **抗病毒药** Antiviral Drug
208. **退烧药** Febrifuge/Antipyretic
209. **特效药** Specific Medicine
210. **法匹拉韦** Favipiravir
211. **可利霉素** Carrimycin
212. **磷酸氯喹** Chloroquine Phosphate
213. **瑞德西韦** Remdesivir
214. **止痛药** Anodyne
215. **抗疟药** Anti-malaria Drug
216. **抗晕动病药物** Anti-motion Sickness Pill
217. **阿司匹林** Aspirin
218. **环丙沙星** Ciprofloxacin
219. **地塞米松** Dexamethasone
220. **安眠药** Sleeping Pill

## （九）常用物品

### （Ⅸ）Common Items

221. **红外体温测量仪** Infrared Thermometer
222. **体温枪 / 体温计** Thermometer
223. **消毒液** Disinfectant / Antiseptic Solution
224. **酒精消毒液** Alcohol-Based Disinfectant
225. **N95 口罩 / 医用外科口罩** N95 Mask / Surgical Mask
226. **防护服** Protective Suit
227. **护目镜** Goggles

228. **一次性手套** Disposable Gloves
229. **标签纸 / 贴纸** Label Paper / Stickers
230. **采样管** Sampling Tube
231. **鼻咽拭子** Nasopharyngeal Swab
232. **检测试剂** Testing Reagent
233. **采血针** Blood Lancet
234. **采血管** Vacutainer
235. **医疗垃圾桶** Medical Waste Bin
236. **杀虫剂** Insecticide
237. **执法记录仪** Body-Worn Camera
238. **耦合剂** Coupling Medicament
239. **驱虫剂** Repellent
240. **避蚊胺** DEET
241. **心电图** ECG
242. **B 超** B-scan Ultrasonography
243. **心电监护仪** Cardiac Monitor

## （十）旅行医学相关名称

## （X）Travel Medicine-related Names

244. **旅行者** Traveler
245. **评估** Assessment
246. **健康咨询** Health Consultation
247. **健康评估** Health Evaluation
248. **高原反应** High Altitude Reaction
249. **流行病学调查** Epidemiological Investigation
250. **疫苗接种** Vaccination
251. **麻疹 - 腮腺炎 - 风疹疫苗** MMR Vaccine

**252. 卡介苗** BCG Vaccine
**253. 黄热病疫苗** Yellow Fever Vaccine
**254. 流脑疫苗** Meningitis Vaccine
**255. 白喉－百日咳－破伤风疫苗** DPT Vaccine
**256. 口服脊髓灰质炎疫苗** OPV Vaccine
**257. 蚊子叮咬** Mosquito Bites
**258. 体格检查** Physical Examination
**259. 疫苗接种证书** Vaccination Certificate
**260. 旅行前** Pre-travel
**261. 旅行后** Post-travel
**262. 预防措施** Precaution
**263. 预防药物** Preventive Drug
**264. 心理咨询** Psychology Consultation
**265. 旅行医疗门诊部** Travel Healthcare Clinic
**266. 旅行计划** Travel Itinerary
**267. 旅行者腹泻** Travelers' Diarrhea
**268. 倒时差** Jetlag
**269. 高原病** Altitude-Illness
**270. 晕动病** Motion Sickness
**271. 意外伤害** Accidental Injury
**272. 日晒** Sun Exposure
**273. 水肺** Scuba
**274. 医疗旅游** Medical Tourism
**275. 回国探亲访友** Immigrants Returning Home to Visit Friends or Relatives
**276. 邮轮旅游** Cruise Ship Travel
**277. 航空旅行** Air Travel

## (十一)其他相关词语和短语

## (XI) Other Related Words and Phrases

**278. 国际关注的突发公共卫生事件**
Public Health Emergency of International Concern (PHEIC)

**279. 突发公共卫生事件** Public Health Emergency

**280. 入境口岸** Port of Entry

**281. 第一入境点** First Point of Entry

**282. 快速通道** Fast Lane/Track

**283. 一米线**
One Meter Spacing in Line (to wait in line at an interval of 1 meter)

**284. 二维码 / 条形码 / 采样码**
QR Code / Bar Code / Sampling Code

**285. 低、中、高风险地区**
Low-, Medium-, High-Risk Regions

**286. 情况说明材料** Factsheet

**287. 戴口罩** Wear a mask

**288. 勤洗手** Wash your hands often

**289. 室内空气流通** Indoor Ventilation

**290. 保持安全距离** Keep safe distance

**291. 避开人群** Avoid crowds

**292. 疫区** Infected Area

**293. 行李、货物和邮包** Luggage, Cargos and Parcels

**294. 检疫处理** Quarantine Treatment

**295. 消毒** Disinfection

**296. 鹅颈结式封扎** Gooseneck Knot Tying

**297. 健康申报** Health Declaration

**298. 体温监测** Body Temperature Monitoring

**299. 医学巡查** Medical Inspection

**300. 医学排查** Medical Screening

**301. 染疫** Pathogen Infection

**302. 染疫嫌疑** Suspected Pathogen Infection

**303. 飞机通风量** Aircraft Ventilation

**304. 流行病学** Epidemiology

**305. 诊断学** Diagnostics

**306. 病理学** Pathology

**307. 潜伏期** Incubation/Latent Period

**308. 感染率 / 发病率 / 病死率**

Infection Rate / Incidence Rate/ Fatality Rate

**309. 飞沫传播** Droplet Transmission

**310. 隐性感染**

Covert / Silent / Inapparent / Subclinical Infection

**311. 交叉感染** Cross Infection

**312. 二代病例** Second-Generation Cases

**313. 基础性疾病** Underlying Medical Conditions

**314. 并发症** Complications

**315. 临床表现** Clinical Manifestations

**316. 临床症状** Clinical Symptoms

**317. 核酸检测** Nucleic Acid Testing (NAT)

**318. 假阴性 / 阳性** False Negative / Positive

**319. 疫苗接种** Vaccination

**320. 抗体检测** Antibody Testing

**321. 基因测序** Gene Sequencing

**322. 职业暴露** Occupational Exposure

**323. 妨害国境卫生检疫罪**

Crime of jeopardizing border quarantine security